From Residency   to Reality

From Residency

to Reality

Patricia A. Hoffmeir
Senior Vice-President, Physician Services/Partner
Garofolo, Curtiss & Company
Ardmore, Pennsylvania

Jean Astolfi Bohner
Owner, Writing at Work
Assistant Professor of English
University of Delaware
Newark, Delaware

McGraw-Hill Book Company
New York   St. Louis   San Francisco   Colorado Springs   Oklahoma City
Auckland   Bogotá   Caracas   Hamburg   Lisbon   London   Madrid
Mexico   Milan   Montreal   New Delhi   Panama   Paris   San Juan
São Paulo   Singapore   Sydney   Tokyo   Toronto

NOTICE

Medicine is an ever-changing science. As new research and clinical experience broaden our knowledge, changes in treatment and drug therapy are required. The editors and the publisher of this work have checked with sources believed to be reliable in their efforts to provide drug dosage schedules that are complete and in accord with the standards accepted at the time of publication. However, readers are advised to check the product information sheet included in the package of each drug they plan to administer to be certain that the information contained in these schedules is accurate and that changes have not been made in the recommended dose or in the contraindications of administration. This recommendation is of particular importance in connection with new or infrequently used drugs.

1 2 3 4 5 6 7 8 9 0 DOC DOC 9 8 2 1 0 9 8 7

ISBN-0-07-029212-4

This book was set in Souvenir by the McGraw-Hill Book Company Publishing Center in cooperation with Monotype Composition Company. The editors were William Day and Julia White; the cover was designed by Edward R. Schultheis; the production supervisor was Elaine Gardenier.
R. R. Donnelley was the printer and binder.

Library of Congress Cataloging-in-Publication Data

Hoffmeir, Patricia A.
    From residency to reality.

    Bibliography: p.
    Includes index.
    1. Medicine—Practice. 2. Job hunting. I. Bohner, Jean Astolfi. II. Title. [DNLM: 1. Career Choice. 2. Internship and Residency. 3. Professional Practice.
W 87 H711f]
R728.H64   1987   610.69'52   87-26160
ISBN 0-07-029212-4

CONTENTS

Dedication

To my mother, who would have been proud of me, and to my husband and daughters, who are proud of me.

P.A. Hoffmeir

To Chris, Russ, and Kate

J. A. Bohner

ACKNOWLEDGMENTS

We would like to thank the many people who have helped in the preparation of this book:

John J. Coury, Jr., M.D., and Dennis O'Leary, M.D., discussed with us their views of today's changing medical environment. Drawing on her years of experience in health care, Sandra Grossman offered valuable suggestions for portions of the manuscript, especially for Chapter X. Also for Chapter X, we are greatly indebted to Thomas Battles for sharing with us what he learned in his many years of medical practice management. David Nash, M.D., M.B.A., helped us solve the puzzle of managed care. Our editor, Bill Day of McGraw-Hill, kept us on track. His advice and suggestions have made this a better book.

Richard Bonfiglio, M.D., has carefully read every chapter and suggested changes from a physician's point of view. His help on Chapter IX was invaluable. We can never repay Rick, not only for his time, but also for his belief in our idea.

Although they wish to remain anonymous, we would like to recognize the many physicians and health-care executives who shared their insights and experiences with us. This book would not have been possible without their help.

Finally, we would like to thank Pete, Lynn, Lauren, Christine, Christopher, Russ, Kate for their support and encouragement, for their understanding when we couldn't be there, and for listening; Christine, Russ, and Kate for editing portions of the manuscript; and Pete for pouring the wine.

FOREWORD

Because of day-to-day practice constraints and specialization, physicians just completing their medical school education never know more about recent medical technological advances than at this time in their careers. But they never know less about practice issues.

Technological advances make practicing medicine more exciting and rewarding, but business constraints can limit opportunities for recent graduates—unless they are prepared. Being prepared to cope with the business of medicine is particularly important in those geographic areas and medical fields with physician oversupply.

Most medical students, however, are not being prepared for the nonclinical aspects of medicine. Paucity of teaching in medical schools and residencies about actual medical practice makes this book an invaluable preparation for medical students and residents approaching the practice of medicine.

In the past it was possible for physicians to establish a practice by hanging out a shingle. Physicians finishing residencies who would prefer just to practice medicine without worrying about so-called business now usually find this impossible. Recent developments, such as the promulgation of patient consumerism over the last three decades and increased government and insurance industry regulation, have greatly complicated this process.

These forces have, in turn, led to increased medical competition and even to the development of brand new styles and settings for medical practices, such as HMOs and PPOs. Even finding a stable position can be difficult, and changing jobs is still more complex. These changes are an unfortunate development but a reality in medicine in the 1980s and beyond.

The pace of change in the business of medicine easily rivals technological advances. Preparing not only for the present business climate but also for future developments, especially for people entering medical practice, is imperative. With decades ahead to consider, changes physicians can expect during their practice life are great—both in technology and in business. Physicians must therefore analyze practice opportunities in the same fashion that they evaluate patients through diagnostic testing.

The first step is establishing a network during medical school and residency that will facilitate identification of practice opportunities. Physicians also must develop the ability to promote themselves through appropriate interview skills and other basic interpersonal skills. Doing so requires an adroit sense of one's abilities and needs.

After establishing a practice, physicians must have enough business sense and ability to achieve the economic success that should follow their clinical achievement. Achieving this success requires an understanding of practice constraints, interaction with other professions, and an understanding of marketing needs.

Most physicians learn in the nonclinical areas of medicine through experience, both good and bad. By exploring the business of medical practice, this book will help medical students and residents enhance their practice opportunities and reduce the likelihood of significant business missteps.

Richard Paul Bonfiglio, M.D.
Medical Director and Residency Program Director
Schwab Rehabilitation Center

Chairman of Physical Medicine and Rehabilitation
Mount Sinai Hospital Medical Center
Chicago

PREFACE

Medical training provides you with excellent clinical skills but does little to prepare you for the realities of having to find a job and of practicing in the modern world of "big business" medicine. In the "good old days," M. Deities finished training, decided where they wanted to practice, and hung out their shingles—fairly certain of financial success. Although technology has made modern medicine an exciting field to be in and although practicing medicine still offers many rewards, the certainties of the good old days are gone. Because of intense competition for jobs and because of the changing demands of providing health care, physicians can no longer rest on their credentials. Candidates for jobs are often turned down because they are not good "team players" or because they project an inappropriate or unprofessional image in the interview.

Like other professionals, most physicians now have to market themselves. But many young physicians, and even older ones moving from their present jobs, have almost no idea about how to search for jobs that will satisfy their personal and professional needs, about how to assess their chances of getting the jobs they want, about how to get the jobs once they have identified them, or about negotiating their contracts once they get the jobs.

They also seldom understand what is happening in the business aspects of medicine. Modern medicine is big business. It is profit oriented. As a result, if they are to survive financially, physicians have to be entrepreneurial. If they are not, they may end up like the family medicine specialist who after more than ten years of practice still lives in a two-bedroom apartment over his office and is still paying off medical school debts—in spite of working day and night. He charges $15 for each visit, nothing more. All procedures, for example, are included in the $15. He says, "I'm a doctor, not a businessman. I'm too busy to bother about charges. Fifteen dollars sounds fair to me." It may sound fair, but it is hardly realistic. His wife finally called in a practice management consultant to help him develop a profitable practice.

This book is intended to help you understand the realities of the world of modern medicine and to help you make your way through that world successfully. It began as a how-to book for physicians coming out of residency and looking for their first jobs. But as we talked to medical students, residents, experienced physicians, and medical school deans and counselors, we discovered that many of you are so caught up in the demands of your training that you do not have a clear picture of what is happening outside your medical schools or training programs. And we also realized that you need to look carefully at some of these realities as you choose your residency. So we wrote Chapters I and II, "Looking at the Future of Medicine," and "Getting Started in Residency."

Neither of these chapters is intended to be definitive. Chapter I is an overview, a summary of some of the current trends in providing health care in the United States. Chapter II discusses some of the problems in choosing a residency and offers advice about how you might solve them. It also suggests more detailed sources of information which you might turn to for help in making such an important decision about your future.

Because beginning to build your network in medicine early in your training is such an integral part of your success as a physician, we devoted an entire chapter, Chapter III, to the areas beyond clinical competency that you will be judged on when you apply for a job. Chapters IV, V, and VI are intended to help you set practical and realistic goals for the kind of job you want, to help you avoid frustrating and time-consuming job shopping, to help you choose a job that will be satisfying.

Chapters VII and VIII offer advice about how to get the job you want. Many physicians do not know where or how to begin their job searches. Also, because they are not business oriented, they are often unaware of some of the pitfalls of interviewing. Chapter VII suggests various methods of marketing yourself, and Chapter VIII tells you how to interview successfully.

Because contract negotiation has become so complicated, with so many variables that you need to be aware of, we added Chapter IX to help you avoid some of the more common mistakes that young physicians often make in negotiating—or in failing to negotiate—their contracts. Chapter X discusses some of the problems that you will have to solve if you want to set up and manage your own practice.

We also realized that because physicians who want to change jobs must go through many of the same steps in their job searches that people coming out of residency do, they could profit from much of the advice in this book. To help them further, we added Chapter XI which discusses some of the additional problems involved in changing jobs. Chapters IX, X, and XI are intended only to raise questions and to suggest possible answers, not to provide final answers. Many books and articles contain more detailed information about solving these problems. Also, in all three of these areas, we suggest that you get professional help from search consultants, attorneys, accountants, and practice management consultants.

Much of the information—especially about networking, assessing your needs and your value, marketing yourself, and interviewing—comes out of Patti Hoffmeir's many years of experience as a physician search consultant. The idea for the book grew from her counseling of physicians involved in job searches, helping them to define the kinds of jobs they would be happy in and to prepare for interviews and to negotiate their contracts. Concerned that the physicians she worked with had little training for the difficult task of finding jobs, she said, "Clearly, no one is preparing young physicians for life after residency. I want to write down all the advice that I give them so they'll have a guide for their real-life career decisions just as they have guides for their medical decisions." Jean Bohner, a free-lance writer who has written about health-care recruiting and health and fitness, agreed to help her put together a how-to manual for physicians searching for their first jobs.

But as we got into the project, we realized that a greater need existed, that physicians at all levels need advice about dealing with the realities of the medical marketplace. In doing research, we were unable to find one book that addresses all the problems of establishing yourself in practice—from choosing a residency to changing jobs. So we decided to write this book.

In gathering information, we relied primarily upon interviews and talks with medical students, residents, practicing physicians, physician administrators, people involved in medical education, hospital administrators, health-care consultants, and patients. Because all but a few of these people wished to be anonymous, we decided not to name anyone. Also, when people who might be recognized by title or specialty or location felt strongly about remaining anonymous, we disguised them further by changing the specialty to a similar one or by changing the location. For example, the Connecticut OB/GYN we quote in the first chapter is actually from a comparable place in the Midwest.

We also relied on a great deal of printed material—everything from books such as Paul Starr's *The Social Transformation of American Medicine* to conference notes. Because we wanted the book to be informal, readable, and accessible and because many of our facts are fairly common ones that appear in a variety of sources but just have not been collected and organized in one place, we did not footnote information. Instead, we have provided a bibliographical essay which contains the primary sources of information for each chapter.

As you read some of the examples we use to illustrate important issues, you may find yourself saying, "No way! This can't be true. Nobody would do that." But some real physician did. Use these examples to capitalize on the experiences of other physicians, to help you avoid some of the more common mistakes physicians make as they try to establish themselves in practice. Making career decisions is a rigorous and demanding process. We hope that you find this book useful and informative and that it will help smooth your path from residency to the reality of practicing medicine in a rapidly changing medical environment. Good luck.

Wilmington, Delaware
June 1987

From Residency   to Reality

Chapter I

Looking at the Future of Medicine

A fair conclusion is that, by the abandonment of blood-letting, a useful measure of treatment was given up. . . . The time will come (and that ere long, for it is now foreshadowed) when it will have its proper rank among therapeutic agencies.

Dr. Austin Flint, *Medicine of the Future*, 1886

Austin Flint, an American physician addressing the British Medical Society, also cautioned against specialization and its possible detrimental effect on the profession of medicine as a whole. Predicting the future is a tricky business. But in the calm and relatively stable world of the late nineteenth century when God was in His heaven and all was right with the world, Flint could point confidently to the "glorious future" of the medical profession.

In the turmoil of the late twentieth century, predictors of the future cannot be so confident. Five years ago, for example, futurists were saying that by 1990 health care would be managed by about twenty nationwide health-care providers. Now, both John J. Coury, Jr., president of the American Medical Association, and Dennis O'Leary, president of the Joint Commission on Accreditation of Hospitals, disagree with that prediction. And Jeff Goldsmith, president of Health Futures, Inc., and author of *Can Hospitals Survive*, says that "Supermeds" are out.

But one thing is sure: The physician as God is dead. Only the physician as professional businessperson or as employee will survive. As one Boston physician said, "God doesn't have to advertise, and He sure as hell doesn't have to try to figure out which form or regulation applies to which procedure."

As power shifts from the providers of health care to the payers, physicians are finding themselves with less and less autonomy. For example, the same computers that allow physicians to make miraculous diagnoses are allowing the government and health-care corporations to establish huge longitudinal data bases which they will use to set nationwide standards for medical treatment. Using a computed average length of hospital stay for each specific diagnosis, the government is already applying standards of this type, diagnostic-related groupings (DRGs), to determine how much it will reimburse hospitals for Medicare and Medicaid patient visits. Many people believe that DRGs are only a small taste of the future.

As patients become consumers, thereby relegating physicians to the general service industry the American public so mistrusts, physicians are losing the enormous prestige and power they have traditionally commanded. As the patient pool shrinks as a result of the large numbers of physicians entering the profession and as inflation and malpractice insurance drive up the cost of practicing medicine, physicians are no longer finding medicine the open sesame to wealth that it has been.

Modern physicians are caught in a series of paradoxes. The public expects physicians to be warm humanists and at the same time brilliant scientists. The integration of C. P. Snow's two cultures, the humanities and the sciences, is one of the great dilemmas of modern life. Yet we see nothing out of the ordinary in our rather casual expectation that physicians, at least, can solve the problem. And now physicians are expected to be successful entrepreneurs as well. Christine Cassell, chief of general internal medicine at the University of Chicago and president of the Society for Health and Human Values, said recently, "There's a lot of pressure for the profession to change, to become more cost-effective and efficient. But if we don't also become more humanistic, we will be in big trouble."

Physicians are being told that to survive they will have to learn to compete for patients both with each other and with their sometimes antagonists, hospitals. Goldsmith calls metropolitan areas such as New York and Los Angeles "medical combat zones." How are physicians to compete for their share of the market? By cooperating—with each other and with hospitals.

Physicians are also being told to cut costs. The length of time they spend with each patient, the number and kinds of tests they order, their referrals to specialists and to hospitals—all are under close scrutiny from the groups paying for their service. At the same time, physicians live with the constant threat of malpractice. The length of time physicians spend with each patient, the number and kinds of tests they order, referrals to specialists and to hospitals—all are under close scrutiny from the people receiving their service.

With its promise of independence, prestige, and economic security, of a life spent in close, helping relationships with patients, the golden city that beckoned at the end of your long and arduous medical education has disappeared. Many young physicians leaving residency say that medicine is not the dream they had of it when they decided to become physicians.

A family medicine specialist on the West Coast says that as a poor, black youth growing up on a farm in Mississippi, he had as a role model the community general practitioner. So, hoping that he too could help people, could make them well, he got himself to medical school. Singled out for his excellent clinical and diagnostic skills, he was steered to internal medicine and was advised to consider a subspecialty. "When I looked around, everything seemed too cold and too clinically oriented. I wanted long-term patient relationships with whole families, so I chose family medicine—even though it meant less money, longer hours, and poor coverage. My mentors didn't much like my decision. But it was as close as I could come to satisfying my ideals."

What happened to the dream?

Health care in the United States has become big business. We spend more on health care than we do on defense, more than ten percent of our gross national product. "Health-care services" has become the "health-care industry." And the catch phrase these days is "the bottom line is profits." The introduction of Medicare and Medicaid into the health-care system in the 1960s made providing health care a lucrative business.

Responding to the traditional image of physicians' need to practice medicine without restraints if they are to do their best work, Congress voted the money but no ceiling on fees. Responding to the same image, traditional insurers also paid the physician's "customary fee" without asking if the fee was a reasonable one.

The result was an unprecedented spiral in the amount of money available for health care and in the amount of health care being provided—for, of course, the more tests, the more procedures, the more hospital beds filled, the more money.

To keep up with expansion and to meet the nation's perceived medical needs, government also underwrote the construction of hospitals, the development of new medical schools, the expansion of old ones, and some of the costs of medical education. Seeing that seemingly boundless green pasture, corporations moved in. Medicare and Medicaid began in 1965, and by 1968 the first of the large for-profit corporations, Hospital Corporation of America, was formed. And corporations brought to the largely independent and decentralized health-care field the same consolidation and cost accounting and management policies that they applied to their other for-profit ventures. Nonprofit, or tax-exempt, hospitals soon followed their lead (with the result that some not-for-profits are now more profitable than the for-profits).

As they saw profits going to hospitals for tests and procedures they could do themselves, many physicians began to set up their own labs and clinics, creating "docs in a box," ambulatory care centers (ACCs) and urgent care centers (UCCs). Although they were occasionally set up in competition with hospitals, no one seemed to notice or to care—there was plenty for everyone.

In the midst of this expansion and prosperity, another movement, the counterculture movement, was taking shape that would profoundly alter society's attitude toward health care. As Paul Starr, Princeton sociologist, says in *The Social Transformation of American Medicine,* there was in the late 1960s and early 1970s a "deepening ambivalence about medicine in the entire society." The women's movement, for example, attacked the medical profession as sexist and sickness-oriented and demanded that women have more say in what happened to them. At the same time, women were joining the profession in large numbers.

The culture as a whole became more interested in "natural cures" and, more important, in "natural prevention." We turned to Adele Davis and Euell Gibbons for cures for everything from insomnia to varicose veins. The young suburban mother who in the early nineteen sixties was severely criticized by her family and friends when she threw away many of the pediatrician's prescriptions for antibiotics, saying that she knew more about her children than the physician did, suddenly became a wise and strong mother. But when the children were "really sick," she demanded that the pediatrician cure them—immediately.

Alternative forms of treatment gained credibility—acupuncture, massage, faith healing, nutritional counseling, what we have come to call holistic medicine. We began to insist on looking at the whole person. One director of a health and exercise center said, "For too long we have said to the physician, 'Here, you take the body'; to the psychiatrist, 'Here, you take the mind'; to the clergyman, 'Here, you take the spirit.' But we're coming to see that people don't split up that easily." Calvinist America with its blind faith in scientific progress was finally saying, "Wait. Where is this leading? What does it mean?" Quality of life also became an important consideration. And, in the process of all this questioning, the traditional authority of the physician was eroding.

But, again, as long as there was plenty for everyone, no one paid much attention. Then one day there was no longer plenty for everyone. As medical costs rose higher and higher, the people paying those costs began to notice. Lee Iacocca, for example, in trying to bail out Chrysler, discovered that Chrysler was spending more for medical insurance than it was for steel. The government (which by now picks up more than forty percent of the nation's health-care bill) and the employers who paid their employees' medical insurance began to look for ways to cut back. By the late 1970s, cost containment had arrived.

Although the idea of health maintenance organizations (HMOs) has been around for more than fifty years, they were not a major factor in the health-care industry until the middle seventies, when their growth was spurred by the government's and industry's efforts to stem the rising cost of medical care. By June 1985, the six largest HMOs in the country enrolled over eight million people—even though most people do not know what they are. (See Fig. 1.)

Because HMOs operate under advance payment for health care rather than under fee-for-service health care, their annual subscriber fees are based on average rather than actual cost of treatment. The result is a strong incentive to hold down the number of referrals to specialists, of authorized procedures, and of hospital admissions. Many large HMOs also limit the amount of time the physician spends with each patient.

All this is supposed to represent savings to third-party payers, up to twenty-five percent a year. Many corporation benefits managers believe HMOs to be so cost effective that they compel new employees to join HMOs rather than give them the option of electing traditional coverage such as that provided by Blue Cross/Blue Shield.

The American Medical Association (AMA), however, questions the

What is an HMO?

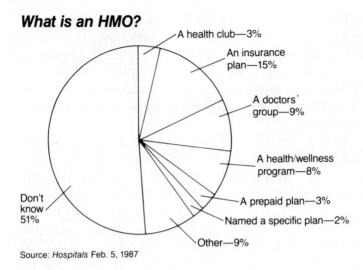

A health club—3%

An insurance plan—15%

A doctors' group—9%

A health/wellness program—8%

A prepaid plan—3%

Named a specific plan—2%

Other—9%

Don't know 51%

Source: *Hospitals* Feb. 5, 1987

Figure 1

assumption that HMOs are more economical. Coury says, "For the first year it has been found that costs may be less, but after the first year costs are about the same." And a Johnson & Higgins 1986 survey of 1500 corporations in thirty-six states confirms Coury's statement: Seventy percent of the corporations offering HMOs reported that HMO rates were as high or higher than those of private insurers.

Whether HMOs are more cost effective than other plans or not, the fact that they are perceived to be suggests that they will continue to affect the way health care is provided in the future. At least their concept of managed health care and the government's institution of DRGs, the very idea of national standards of treatment, seem to have permanently changed the provision of health care in the United States.

Many group health insurers, to meet the competition of HMOs while at the same time allowing clients to choose their own physicians, have formed preferred provider organizations (PPOs). Essentially the PPO acts as an agent between employers and the medical community. The insurer negotiates lower health-care costs for the employer while guaranteeing a steady supply of patients to the medical community.

Physicians are also turning to PPOs to head off competition from

HMOs. Coury says that in some communities, to protect themselves, physicians are banding together to form PPO "paper" arrangements so that when large third-party insurers such as CIGNA come into the community, the insurers will have to turn to them as an already established group able to provide the necessary array of patient services.

One of the problems of PPOs, the difficulty of assessing their quality, is currently being addressed by the American Association of Preferred Provider Organizations (AAPPO). The AAPPO plans to offer by mid-1987 a voluntary credentialing program for PPOs, which will examine their "provider selection, benefit design, quality assurance guidelines, utilization review protocols, and financial solvency."

Another response of the medical community to competition for patients is the formation of independent practice associations (IPAs), a type of HMO in which member physicians are paid a yearly standard fee for each member patient. Like PPOs, IPAs allow physicians the autonomy of private practice from their own offices. But because patients prepay for treatment, holding down costs is in the physicians' best interests. (For a detailed discussion of HMOs, PPOs, and IPAs, see Chapter V.)

Current trends suggest a movement away from large, nationwide HMOs and the government's use of DRGs. The Johnson & Higgins survey shows that PPOs are generally more cost-effective than HMOs and that many employers plan to add PPOs to their benefit options. Also, a joint survey by the American Hospital Association and Arthur Andersen & Co., the results of which were reported at the February 1987 annual meeting of the American Hospital Association (AHA), predicts that although "deficit reductions will continue to motivate most government health care financing decisions," the government will turn to prepaid health care through HMOs and PPOs rather than continue to use measures such as DRGs, primarily because such measures are so difficult to administer.

Employees as well as employers and the government like the idea of prepaid plans. In most prepaid plans, employees know exactly what their share in the cost of their health care will be. There are no surprises and no huge bills. For each office visit, for example, the fixed copay rate might be as low as one to five dollars. Also, employees do not have to worry about filling out insurance forms and often prescription medicines are covered as well as treatment. In prepaid plans, employees have less choice than in traditional plans but lower costs.

Physicians themselves are not so enthusiastic about prepaid plans or about the basic concept of health-care management. The loss of autonomy and the regimentation go against the tradition of the physician as independent professional. In addition to chafing under the restrictions of alternative health care delivery, many physicians dislike the loss of long-term patient contact. One internist-nephrologist in New York City is leaving a large HMO because "I have to see a patient every ten minutes. If a patient needs dialysis, I never see him again. I don't have any real relationship with my patients." A Boston pediatrician is leaving her HMO because "the whole business atmosphere really gets to me. Sometimes the problem isn't going to be solved by prescribing medication. I need to talk to the parents about nontraditional medical problems. The parents of a dehydrated eighteen-month-old who is dehydrated because he's not eating don't need medicine; they need counseling. How can I provide it in my allotted twelve minutes?"

Although most physicians do not like the idea, prepaid health care and health-care management will most likely dominate the future of medicine. Certainly, being a part of some kind of group, no matter how loosely organized, would seem to be the answer to many of the problems that physicians will have in the future. For example, according to Coury, getting malpractice insurance in some states is becoming virtually impossible unless the physician is associated with a group. Also, when asked why he became a member of a large health-care plan after almost thirty years in private practice, a Connecticut OB/GYN answered, "It was join or lose patients. Or advertise. I'll never reconcile myself to doctors on TV hawking their services—like people selling cars."

In mentioning advertising, the physician touched on one of the central problems in the future of medicine: the decreasing supply of patients and increasing supply of physicians. Many things are credited with or blamed for—depending on your point of view—the decreasing supply of patients. Cost-containment policies, of course, head the list with fewer procedures, fewer referrals, fewer hospital admissions, and shorter stays for those admitted. Also society's move to wellness, to preventive medicine has certainly contributed to the fall-off. Goldsmith says that "it is becoming increasingly apparent that everyone can have enormous impact on his or her own health status by proper exercise, diet, and the avoidance of known health hazards such as smoking."

Many people predict that the patient pool will stabilize. The graying of America will mean a larger percentage of the population will need health care. Older people are sicker. The growth of fields such as physiatry and sports medicine will bring in more patients. Earlier, physiatrists' patients would have either died or gone into some sort of chronic care facility. Sports medicine physicians' patients would have lived with their tennis elbows and bad knees.

The increasing supply of physicians also shows signs of stabilizing. It is true that the expansion of the medical schools in the 1960s and 1970s has brought unprecedented numbers of people into the profession. In the thirty years from 1960 to 1990, it is predicted that the number of physicians for every one hundred thousand people will increase by almost one hundred, from one hundred forty-eight to two hundred forty-five. By 1990 almost half of the people practicing medicine in the United States will have entered the profession since 1978.

But for the first time in recent years, admissions to medical school are going down. The "bad press" that medicine has been getting seems to be one reason. A recent Cornell graduate left premed for engineering because he did not like what he was hearing about medicine: "Why spend all that time—eight or ten years of working nights, thirty-six hour days—and all that money just to come out and maybe have to go to work for somebody else? At least now I'm not in debt, and I can go skiing on weekends if I want to."

Another reason is that new technology is offering more options for people who are bright and good at science and mathematics. Coury believes that in the past medicine was one of the few places available for these people. Now, however, fields such as computer science, biochemistry, and biomedical engineering are drawing people away from medicine. While she was a premed student at Swarthmore College, one young woman found that she really did not like the idea of dealing with old, sick people even though she liked the idea of helping people be healthy. In exploring career possibilities, she discovered biomedical engineering. She's now working on the design and manufacture of artificial joints.

Not everyone agrees that the change in the physician-patient ratio is a real problem for the profession. Many people, such as O'Leary, believe that there is not an oversupply of physicians, just a maldistribution. So the change will, in effect, bring quality health care to areas such as remote rural towns and poor urban centers where it has been noticeably absent.

Also, who would argue that the loss of people like the Cornell and Swarthmore engineers is a tragedy for medicine? The person who wants his weekends free and a large dollar return on his time would probably not have made a very good doctor. And the person who dislikes interacting with sick people certainly would not. Ten years ago they both might have stayed in the profession because they would not have seen anywhere else to go.

Another change that is resulting from the changed ratio is what some people are calling the *rehumanization* of medicine. Physicians and hospitals are having to cultivate patients to build their patient pool, or even to keep it. So physicians are spending more time with their patients. And the house call has returned—for a price, to be sure. One Washington, D.C., physician charges $100 for each house call. The prediction is that house calls will once again become part of the physician's routine and that they will become more reasonably priced.

Another factor in the rehumanization of medicine is the large numbers of women entering the profession—just about a third of entering medical students are female. Women physicians are likely to be more empathetic and more willing to listen to and spend time with their patients. They are also more likely to have good relations with ancillary staff. In the new world of medicine, these qualities, which did not matter much when the physician was God, can only improve the quality of modern health care because cooperation is being seen more and more as the key to survival.

Rather than compete for patients, hospitals and physicians are moving together to solve the problems of providing cost-effective and efficient but, at the same time, health-effective and humane care. Traditionally, this kind of cooperation has been difficult to achieve because, as Goldsmith says, the relative isolation of their practices has often made it "difficult to get physicians to view the medical needs of the community as a whole." Now, however, they are being forced out of isolation and into the community.

Also, hospitals often saw physicians as adversaries, particularly when physicians began offering many of the same services, such as laboratory and x-ray services. But economic pressures have made the protection of the hospitals' referral bases increasingly important. Obviously, the size and type of this base is closely related to the number and quality of doctors associated with the hospital. To keep beds filled, many hospitals recruit physicians, paying them guaranteed incomes and giving them office space in return for admissions. No matter how state-of-the-art its equipment, a hospital cannot survive without "good docs." Conversely, good docs need good colleagues and good equipment.

One sign of the times is that the American Foundation of Health Care Executives (AFHCE) offers a two-day seminar called "Optimizing Medical Staff Relationships: Building Understanding, Winning Cooperation." The seminar's description says that "healthcare executives and physicians must find innovative ways to work together.... The key to survival and success is cooperation, not competition."

One of the innovative ways hospitals and physicians are working together is through the formation of hospital-physician joint ventures. (The AFHCE also offers a seminar on how to set up and manage a successful joint venture.) These joint ventures are usually for-profit corporations owned by the hospital and the physicians. For example, when a well known teaching hospital with the largest HMO in its city wanted to move into adjacent communities, it found a good community hospital and formed a joint venture with the hospital's for-profit parent company. Together they opened six urgent-care centers. The physicians are credentialed through the teaching hospital and are guaranteed a patient pool, the hospital gets admissions from the centers, the community is provided with excellent health care. And everyone thrives.

Another form of this type of cooperation is the community hospital in which physicians invest as owners. When, for example, downsizing threatened a fine, small community hospital in the suburbs of a Midwest city, a group of physicians in the community bought into the hospital. Again, everyone has profited—the hospital, the physicians, and most of all the community, whose members receive excellent care in a state-of-the-art facility right in the community.

Hospitals themselves are finding that they must work together if they are to survive. All over the country, city hospitals and hospitals in relatively rural areas are either merging or pooling resources to cut out duplication of services and to save money through group purchasing, by combining supply orders. In the Bethlehem, Pennsylvania, area, for example, community leaders, seeing a diminishing market for the area's two hospitals, realized that they had a choice between cut-throat competition or cooperation. Choosing cooperation, they formed Horizon Health System, Inc., in 1985, and the hospitals are now prospering. Hospitals in Rochester, New York, recently did the same thing—coordinating their efforts both to stay alive and to provide better care.

The need for cooperation extends beyond corporations and groups of people. To survive in the modern medical profession, physicians are finding that they must cooperate not only with each other but also with ancillary staff. Residents who shout at nurses or discount the advice of nonphysician medical professionals might find themselves without a position. Recently, a large urban rehabilitation hospital developed a profile of an ideal candidate for a physiatrist-opening on its staff. Of the twenty qualities the hospital is looking for, only four pertain to clinical expertise. And when one of the attendings of a physician candidate was asked in a reference check what he thought about the candidate, he replied, "He's an excellent doctor. But I'd never work with the s.o.b." The candidate did not get the job. As one hospital administrator said, "We're looking for a team player."

Most of you will need to be team players because most of you will choose to be employees of some sort or members of a group practice rather than private practitioners—for many reasons. The chief reason seems to be economic. The average indebtedness of people coming out of residency in 1985 was $30,000. For many that figure was $60,000 to $70,000. Getting loans to set up a practice is becoming more and more difficult—plus getting the loan will probably put you into six-figure indebtedness. Then, inflation, affecting wages to employees and the cost of supplies, equipment, office space, and malpractice insurance, if you get it privately, drive up the cost of maintaining a practice.

When faced with all this and with the specter of a shrinking patient pool, many of you will opt for a guaranteed income. One Texas internal medicine resident, when asked why she was going to work for an ambulatory care center, said, "I know exactly what my base salary will be [she also gets a percentage of receipts], so I know I can get rid of this huge debt that's hanging around my neck like an albatross. And I won't have to dig and scratch for referrals."

Because you did not go into medicine to be businesspeople, many of you will choose to leave paperwork and marketing to administrators. With Medicare, Medicaid, DRGs, and hundreds of different insurance forms, the paperwork in private practice can be overwhelming. The *New England Journal of Medicine* recently reported that administrative costs make up twenty-two percent of the total health-care costs in the United States. The problem is not just the amount of paperwork. It is the fact that if you do not do your charting correctly, you will not be reimbursed for your services. An orthopedics resident at the Hospital of the University of Pennsylvania admitted that charting is a "weak area for some of us. It's a pain in the neck, but it looks like it's here to stay. We'd better get comfortable with it, I guess, for the future of the hospitals and our practices."

Because medicine is now big business, advertising and marketing—even though the AMA fought the idea—are becoming an important component of health care. And medical marketing has itself become big business. Arthur Sturm, president of Sturm Communications Group, Inc., in Chicago, says that a physician in the Chicago area would have to spend at least $40,000 to $50,000 for a basic marketing and advertising campaign. For a small TV campaign, the physician should plan on "upwards of $100,000." Even the AMA offers a seminar called "Marketing Strategies for Private Practice" designed to help physicians "solve problems through the use of a marketing process and proven techniques which are consistent with medical ethics, good taste, and quality service to patients."

After the grueling years of internship and residency, many of you will be too tired even to contemplate "marketing strategies" and a labyrinth of multicopy forms. You will be looking at the quality of your lives—another reason many of you will become employees, even though in doing so you will give up some of your autonomy. As Starr says, many young physicians are so exhausted from their residencies that they choose "freedom *from* the job rather than freedom *in* the job."

Many young physicians are balking at the idea of hundred-hour weeks that leave them no time for themselves or their families. O'Leary, for example, has found that young physicians are more concerned with lifestyle and professional environment than they are with money and autonomy. In his graduation speech at Harvard Medical School in 1984, Mark Wenneker said, "Our careers will not consume our lives. We want to be more than just good doctors. We want to be good parents and spouses as well." One couple in the Southwest joined a large HMO because they planned to have a family and both wanted to be able to work part time so they could take care of their children themselves rather than be "day-care parents."

Both Coury and O'Leary are optimistic about the future of medicine, for one reason because they find young physicians more adaptable to the changes occurring in the profession and more willing to work for positive change than some senior physicians. Many senior physicians share the attitude of the radiologist in his mid-fifties who said, "None of this stuff affects me. I'm going to ride it out for a couple more years and then retire. I'm not worried. My hay is already in the barn."

For those of you whose hay is not yet in the barn, the future is not so bleak as the media would have it, nor is the profession itself so horribly rapacious. Medicine might be different, but it will not necessarily be worse.

For one thing, technology is enabling physicians to perform medical miracles. And it will continue to make medicine a challenging and exciting field. The recent development, for example, of portable magnetic resonance imagers (MRIs) has suddenly made the most sophisticated diagnostic equipment available to large segments of the population. Now, four or five hospitals can pool their resources and buy one MRI, which they can share. Earlier, MRIs were so expensive that only the largest hospitals could afford them.

The government will probably become more and more involved. In 1987, Congress is exploring ways to provide help for people with "catastrophic" medical expenses and to provide quality care for indigents. In fact, bringing good medical care to the poor is one of the central issues in modern medicine. For example, one happy result of the new spirit of cooperation in medicine is Chicago's Partnerships in Health. Under the program, eight city hospitals are joining with the department of public health to improve the quality and accessibility of health care for the city's poor.

Another concern is the growing number of people under the age of sixty-five without any kind of medical insurance. Senator Edward Kennedy of Massachusetts is working on a bill which would require all employers, no matter how small the business, to provide medical coverage to their employees.

Holding down costs will continue to be an issue. A February 1987 survey showed that the major worry of Americans, far ahead of anything else, is the cost of health care. And 1986 inflation studies would tend to support their concern. Although the consumer price index rose only 1.1 percent in 1986, medical costs rose 7.7 percent—more than any other segment of the economy. So the "incorporation" of American medicine will most likely continue.

Even though this incorporation means that you will have to give up some of the traditional "perks" of medicine, it will also offer many of you new opportunities. Health-care corporations need physicians to act as mediators between the corporations and physicians. So some of you will choose to become health-care executives and managers as a way of ensuring excellent medical care for your communities. Some of you will move into hospital or joint-venture administration for the same reasons.

And even though *Medical Economics* (a journal not often found in waiting rooms) may not be publishing many articles about what to do with the hundred thousand you have left after you have made all your other smart investments, the 1986 average income after expenses for U.S. physicians was $113,000. A figure most of you could live with.

And there are some stirrings toward refining malpractice insurance. Some people are asking why it cannot be figured the way automobile insurance is, with high-risk people paying more. As the Connecticut OB/GYN said, "I've never had one malpractice suit in all my years in practice. Why should I pay the same as the jerk eight blocks away who's had about five in the last five years?" Also, some physicians are solving the problem of malpractice insurance by forming their own malpractice insurance companies. Physician-owned companies exist in more than thirty states. Of the money generated each year by malpractice insurance, more than half comes from these companies.

The physician's comment points to another positive result of the changes in medicine: peer review. For a long time, given the independent nature of the profession, physicians were reluctant to do anything about their incompetent or greedy colleagues. But as they saw "quality control" going to people outside the profession, they instituted rigorous peer review boards. Perhaps in the future the media will not be able to portray the physician as money-hungry and power-mad. Everyone knows that the number of "Medicare fraud" and incompetent physicians is very small, that most physicians care about their patients and about providing excellent care more than they do about making money. But God has to be perfect: When God falls it's big news.

Perhaps not being God will not be such a bad thing. Now, if we lived at a time when the gods could be whimsical and capricious, could change themselves into swans and seduce beautiful young girls or start a war because they were jealous, being God might be more appealing. But our God is stern, all-knowing, all-powerful, and perfect. That is a terrible load to carry.

Also, if some of the predictions in this chapter seem depressing, always remember Flint and bloodletting. (Polycythemia had not yet been diagnosed.) Predicting the future of anything is risky. But trying to predict the future of medicine is almost impossible. Large corporations and marketing strategies aside, medicine is not dealing with refrigerators or boxes of cereal. Despite the catch phrase, the bottom line in medicine is not profits. The bottom line in medicine is people.

Chapter II

Getting Started
in Residency

Although the future of medicine is unpredictable, your own future in medicine need not be so unpredictable. You can exercise some control over your medical career. Because your choice of specialty and of where you will do your residency will have such an enormous impact on your future, you need to do careful research and planning before you make a decision that will in large part determine how you spend the rest of your life.

And you need to begin planning early. To get into some of the more competitive programs, you have to do a clerkship at the program at the beginning of your last year in medical school. What is the rush? You may have to apply for the clerkship in your second year.

Many of you, so caught up in the heavy demands of medical school, tend to approach your choice of specialty rather haphazardly, sometimes choosing the specialty of the physician you most admire in medical school. When asked why they chose their particular specialties, residents often say that they picked the specialty of their medical school mentor, someone who offered them guidance and whom they respected and wanted to be like. They thought they could pour themselves into a mold of their role model, only to find later that they did not fit. In deciding on your specialty in this way, you might be one of the lucky ones who end up in a specialty that is ideally suited to you.

But in leaving such an important decision up to chance, you might end up like the two physicians in their middle forties, one a radiologist and one an OB/GYN, whose professional lives provide little reward beyond a monetary one because they made the wrong choice. When someone said to the radiologist, "With all the new developments in radiology, it must be an exciting field to be in," he replied, "I hate it. Most days I wish I could walk out of my office and never come back. I really want to be in family practice, to have long-term relationships with my patients." His reasons for not doing a residency in family practice? "What do I do with four private school tuitions and college out there on the horizon and the houses and...?" When a patient, who had just been given a severe lashing for relatively minor weight gain, asked the OB/GYN, "Do you like your job?" he answered, "I hate it. Mostly all I do is deal with middle-class women whose only problem is that they eat too much. I should be in emergency medicine." His reasons for staying where he is are almost identical with those of the radiologist.

Making a change earlier in your career is not much easier. A young woman resident in OB/GYN chose the specialty primarily because she had heard that more women were needed in OB/GYN and that the field she really wanted, orthopedics, is a tight fraternity, most of whose members are men. Now in her last year of residency, she got as far as interviewing for two positions before withdrawing her candidacy and applying for a residency in orthopedics. Why? "Because I just couldn't go through with it. I can't spend the rest of my life doing something I'm beginning to hate, even though this decision has turned my life upside down. I've had to postpone my wedding. I may have to live about four hundred miles from my fiancé. My parents have to lend me money.

"Not only that, people will always question the change. They'll think I'm not a good decision maker or that I'm just putting off entering the real world of practicing medicine. This was a gutsy decision, not a wishy washy one. But I'll always have to convince people that I didn't make it because I wasn't a good OB/GYN."

Even so, she is more fortunate than the student still in medical school who sees no other choice but to go into general surgery. Early in medical school he worked with a surgeon whom he admired so much that he did many of his rotations in surgery. By his fourth year he has found that, while he still admires his mentor, he does not want to be in general surgery. But he is applying for a residency in it anyway. Why? "I don't have enough experience in other areas—or contacts. Being in this is like being on a ladder where every time you go up a rung the one under it falls away. I want to do more than just cut and sew, but I can't go back. I don't have a safety net, like wealthy parents, under me. I'll just have to hope for the best."

Instead of hoping for the best, you can plan for the best. All through medical school you are trained to gather as much information as you can before you make a decision about how best to treat a patient. You would never even consider ordering a procedure for a patient just because you like the sound of it or because you like the person performing it. Yet, in effect, some of you choose your specialty for those or similar reasons. Obviously, to make a wise decision, you need to gather as much information as you can—about yourself, about the specialties and subspecialties available to you, and about various residency programs.

The best place to begin is with you—with what you like, with what approach to medicine appeals to you the most. Is your initial emphasis on wellness or on sickness? Are you interested in womb-to-the-tomb medicine or in short-term patient relationships? Do you enjoy relationships with peers more than with patients? Your answers to these and similar questions will help you bring into focus the kinds of specialties you might be happy in. Many of you know vaguely how you would answer these questions. But you need more than general answers; you need to look carefully at how you respond to patients and peers, at how you interact with them. You need to look at how you cope with "failure," with death.

If you are drawn to the idea of wellness, of keeping people well rather than making them well and if you want long-term patient relationships, you'll probably turn to such specialties as family medicine, pediatrics, obstetrics and gynecology, occupational medicine, or internal medicine. These are all specialties which call for more than the usual share of empathy and of counseling skills, for a holistic approach to treatment. Often you will treat whole families in what may prove to be long and laborious relationships. As one physician said recently, "It's easy to love the good-natured patients who do what you tell them and pay their bills on time. It's the others that test our commitment." If you think listening to old Mr. Jones, who came in because he has "indigestion," talk about his bed-ridden wife and his children living a thousand miles away is a waste of valuable time or if your response to the mother who overfeeds her child is anger rather than concern, stay away from these specialties.

To stay wellness oriented, even though you may not enjoy intense, personal relationships with patients or if you are more interested in maintaining the health of society at large rather than of individuals, you can go into a field such as public health, general preventive medicine, or infectious diseases. Here you will work with "populations" rather than with people. But if you are irritated by "politicking" and working in and with bureaucracies, look for another specialty.

What if you know you want long-term, helping relationships with patients, if you are interested in holistic treatment, but you are like the physician who said he went into medicine because he wanted to "fix broken people?" You will probably find specialties such as physical medicine and rehabilitation, psychiatry, or some of the subspecialties of internal medicine (rheumatology, for example) the most satisfying. But to be a physiatrist, you'll need to enjoy working as part of a team, with physical therapists, occupational therapists, social workers, and psychologists. To be a psychiatrist, you'll need to enjoy working alone essentially, with little interaction with other physicians.

If you are primarily interested in fixing broken people and you enjoy establishing quick rapport and trust with patients but you do not particularly want long-term patient relationships, you can turn to specialties such as surgery and its subspecialties, emergency medicine, or to many of the subspecialties of internal medicine. But if you know you like to think your way slowly and carefully through a problem, stay away from emergency medicine. If you want quick results, avoid medical oncology.

You may derive greater satisfaction from interacting with your peers than from interacting with patients. If so, you'll most likely be drawn to specialties such as pathology or radiology. But if you want prestige and power, you will not find these specialties particularly satisfying.

You also need to consider many other factors. Do you want a well-ordered life, with fairly regular hours? Dermatology is a possibility; obstetrics is not. Do you need variety to keep you interested? Neurology is a possibility; colon and rectal surgery is not. Is creativity important to you? Plastic surgery is a possibility; emergency medicine is not. Do you enjoy doing procedures and closely analyzing data? Gastroenterology is a possibility; psychiatry is not.

At this point, some of you—considering your projected indebtedness—may be saying, "Who cares about all these things? What I want is to make money, lots of money." Right now, when you are working harder than you ever thought possible and you are living on borrowed money, this attitude might seem appealing. But make sure you look beyond your desire for a good income. Or you may end up like the physician who said, "I'm tired of standing on the sidewalk and having mud splashed on me by all the Mercedes roaring by. I want to be in the driver's seat." He is now an orthopedic surgeon in New York City. He does not enjoy what he does or where he lives. And he drives a Yugo—keeping a Mercedes in the city is "too complicated."

For some of you, the self-consciousness involved in trying to discover what you like and want to do may seem impossible to achieve. As one first-year medical student said, "How do I know if I'm crisis oriented? Anyway, that's not my problem today. Today, my problem is knowing all the bones in the hand and wrist." Actually, "that" is your problem today. While you obviously do not need to choose your specialty today, you do need to begin doing the research that will help you make a wise decision when the time comes to choose a specialty.

And you can do research on yourself. In her informative and helpful book, *How to Choose a Medical Specialty,* Anita Taylor suggests that when you enter medical school, you begin keeping a journal in which you note the subjects, the people, and the clinical areas that interest you the most and *why* they interest you. As you do your rotations, enter what you like most and least about each one and, again, why.

To help you see yourself more clearly, you can also take a personality test such as the Myers-Briggs Type Indicator. The Office of Student Affairs or its equivalent at your school will either administer the test and discuss the results with you or help you find another agency that provides this type of service.

One problem here for many people is that the evidence in the journals and the test results may contradict their private image of themselves. You may see yourself as creative and flexible—in fact, these qualities might be very important to you. What happens when your journal shows that you are drawn to highly structured clinical experiences rather than to open-ended ones? Or when the test indicates that you are methodical rather than creative? If you want a satisfying professional life, this may be the time to reassess your self-image or, at least, to try to reconcile your subjective with your objective image. This is not an easy thing to do at the best of times. When you are experiencing all the stresses of medical school, you may be tempted to ignore the disparity. But dealing with it now can only make your life easier in the future.

Once you know what you enjoy and what you think you want to do, you need to look at what you *can* do. You may have to reconcile the dream with the reality. From the time you were a child, you may have dreamed of being a plastic surgeon. But if you have poor or even mediocre fine motor skills, you really cannot be a plastic surgeon. Ever since you listened to your best friend's parent describe an exciting procedure in ophthalmology, you may have dreamed of being an ophthalmologist. But if you do not have normal color vision, you really cannot be an ophthalmologist.

Listen to your mentors. They know more than you about what the specialty entails. And they may see you more clearly than you see yourself. One medical student wanted to go into surgical oncology. But his mentors pointed out that he was an excellent, acute diagnostician, that he was better with his head than with his hands. So he chose medical oncology instead. Another was considering nephrology. But her mentors told her they thought she established relationships with children more quickly and easily than with adults, especially older adults. So she chose pediatric nephrology instead.

As the competition for residency positions increases, other factors are affecting what you can do. If you are a foreign medical graduate (FMG), you will find some specialties virtually closed to you. You have almost no chance of getting a residency in specialties such as plastic surgery or neurosurgery. Over the last few years, the number of FMGs, both U.S.-citizen (USFMG) and foreign-native (FNFMG), in U.S. residency programs has been declining—by six percent in 1984–1985.

All FMGs must be certified by the Educational Commission for Foreign Medical Graduates (ECFMG). To be certified, you must be affiliated with a medical school listed in the *World Directory of Medical Schools,* pass the Foreign Medical Graduate Examination in the Medical Sciences (FMGEMS) and the ECFMG English test, and prove that you have completed all the educational requirements to practice medicine in the country in which you completed your medical education. (For more detailed information, write ECFMG at 3624 Market Street, Philadelphia, Pennsylvania 19104-2685.)

FMGs who graduate from accredited U.S. undergraduate premedical programs and whose undergraduate work meets the requirements for matriculation into accredited U.S. medical schools may choose the "Fifth Pathway" to give themselves a better chance of getting the specialty they want. If your medical school is listed in the *World Directory of Medical Schools* and if you have completed all the requirements of the school except for internship and/or social work, you may apply to substitute for the internship and/or social work an academic year of supervised clinical training at an approved U.S. medical school. Although you still have to pass the FMGEMS and meet other requirements, a Fifth Pathway certificate gives you much more flexibility in choosing a specialty than an ECFMG certificate does.

While the number of FMGs in residency has been declining, the number of osteopathic physicians has been increasing. Your chances, however, of getting into a competitive specialty are fewer if you are in osteopathic rather than allopathic medicine. But in looking for less competitive specialties, you may find one more suited to you than the one you think you want. A doctor of osteopathy (D.O.), the one who wants to fix broken people, wanted plastic surgery but chose physical medicine and rehabilitation instead. He says, "I'm much happier in physiatry than I would have been in plastic surgery. I like the variety and the emphasis on the whole patient. And I also get to use my basic osteopathic training."

Your grades and your scores on the National Boards, particularly on Part I, are other factors affecting what you can do in medicine. If your grades or scores are low, you will most likely find that the more competitive specialties will be closed to you. So if you want a specialty such as otolaryngology or anesthesiology, which are among the most competitive specialties, you need to pay close attention to grades and board scores. Finishing in the bottom third of your class, no matter how prestigious your undergraduate program, might keep you out of the field you want to work in.

At the same time that you are determining what you want to do and what you can do, you need to be finding out as much as you can about the requirements of each of the specialties and subspecialties. The most obvious place to start is with your rotations. Do not limit yourself to fields you think you might like. Work in as many areas as you can. For example, most of the interns at a good, but certainly not prestigious, hospital in the Middle Atlantic area said they chose the hospital in part because of its central location on the East Coast but primarily because of the variety of clinical experiences available there.

While you are in each rotation, get to know as many of the attendings as you can. Find out as much as you can about what they do, what a typical day is for them, how they feel about their work. Talk to the residents in each area about the same things and about why they chose that specialty. Watch the people in the field. Which ones seem happiest? Why? Which ones seem the most stressed? Why?

Also, read as much as you can about the specialties, look at the journals in each specialty. Read the latest copy of the AMA's annual *Directory of Residency Training Programs,* the "green book." Section I provides information about FMG requirements, appointment to the Armed Services Residency Training Programs, and the National Resident Matching Program (NRMP). In Section II, which discusses the requirements for the accreditation of all specialties, you can read about the type of residency program mandated for each specialty, about the general curriculum you would be following in each one. Section III is a summary of the statistics on graduate medical education in the United States. It lists the number of Post-graduate Year 1 (PGY-1) positions offered in each specialty for the past 3 years, the number of residents on duty in each specialty during the past 3 years, and the number of women, blacks, osteopathic physicians, USFMGs, FNFMGs, and Fifth Pathway FMGs. Studying the statistics might help you assess your chances of getting the specialty you want.

In conjunction with Section III, read the Graduate Medical Education National Advisory Committee (GMENAC) Summary Final Report and its 1982 update by the Department of Health and Human Services. These reports project for the year 1990 the balance between numbers of physicians in each specialty with the need for each specialty. So if you are considering diagnostic radiology, for example, and see a projected surplus of 35 percent, you may want to look at therapeutic radiology, which has a projected shortage of 15 percent.

Once you have determined your own personality profile, see how it matches the personality profiles of specialists in each field. Find copies of Mary McCaulley's *Application of the Myers-Briggs Type Indicator to Medicine and Other Health Professions* or of George Zimney's *Medical Specialty Preference Inventory.* Both discuss the most common personality traits of people in each specialty.

You can also turn to works designed specifically to help you choose your specialty. Taylor's book, in addition to giving general advice about choosing a specialty, discusses each specialty individually. Each section, after a general discussion of the specialty, provides information about available residencies, board certification, supply and projections, economic status and types of practice, and the address and phone number of the academy or college of physicians governing the specialty.

Perhaps the most helpful part of each section is the "Composite Picture" of the specialty, drawn from the responses of 282 physicians. They provided the answers to questions you would certainly ask about each specialty: why choose it, what do they like most and least, what is a typical daily schedule, what abilities and talents are important, what personality traits characterize the people in that specialty, what advice can they give you, what are the future challenges? The section closes with the specialists' top three choices of their specialties' nonclinical aspects which most appeal to them and, perhaps more interesting, with the choices that no one made. Emergency medicine physicians, for example, had variety as the top choice, but no one chose creativity. Also, Taylor does a summary personality profile of the specialists, which you can check yourself against.

Another book is the Pfizer *Guide to Medical Career Opportunities.* It is divided into sections on each specialty, with a physician in the field writing about the pros and cons of the specialty and about such things as kinds of practice settings. Medical students in the throes of making specialty and program choices have themselves written "Answers to the Medical Student's Dilemma: Choosing a Specialty, Selecting a Residency, the Match," published by the American Medical Students Association (AMSA) in the monograph *Pulse.*

Still another source of information is the counseling center or student affairs office at your medical school. Many medical schools have programs specifically designed to help students choose their specialties, assigning them to physician-counselors and setting up career days, when specialists come to talk with students. Jefferson Medical College, for example, has special sessions in which students between their second and third years have an opportunity to talk to alumni in various specialties. Also, each department has a resident advisory committee. You should take advantage of these services—even when you think you cannot fit one more thing into your already overcrowded schedule.

You also need to take a hard look at the future of the specialties you are interested in. While the technological advances in a field may make it particularly exciting, remember that the development of a new test could radically change the nature of the field—as laser surgery did in ophthalmology. If you are going into a field because you are interested in doing a special procedure, technological advances may make the procedure obsolete. And look at your own future in the field. If you concentrate on a procedure that requires steady hands and extremely fine motor skills, will you be able to continue doing the procedure as you get older?

Having found out as much as you can about yourself and about the various specialties, you should have no trouble now picking your specialty. Right? Sometimes. For many of you, the choice will still be difficult because you have to make the choice before you have had a chance to complete your rotations. Over and over again, residents say things like "I might have chosen hematology, for example, but I didn't do a rotation in it until I was already matched." You can, at least in part, avoid this problem by learning all you can about the specialties soon enough to choose early rotations in the ones which you think might be possibilities for you.

Far more difficult is juggling all the variables. A student at school in the Mid-West, for example, found himself drawn in many different directions. He liked the idea of psychiatry, but "a lot of the jocks in med school think psychiatrists are wimps." So he did not seriously consider it. He was attracted to some of the subspecialties of internal medicine because of their intellectual challenge: "When I go to the library, I always pick up the medicine journals first." But he found the amount of death in these subspecialties—"so much death"—too draining emotionally.

In college, he had two knee operations and admired the orthopedic surgeon who treated him. Also, in medical school he thought the orthopedic surgeons he worked with seemed the happiest and most satisfied of all the specialists. But he was interested most of all in preventive medicine and holistic treatment and in working with families.

Narrowing his choice finally to orthopedics and family medicine, he chose orthopedics for two reasons. One, he wanted a family life of his own and thought that in orthopedics he would have more control over his time. Two, because orthopedics is more competitive, he thought that if he decided to do a second residency, moving from orthopedics would be easier than moving to it.

Now in the middle of his residency, he finds that work in prevention of osteoporosis and of sports-related injuries in children is satisfying. But he is seriously considering doing a second residency in either family medicine or psychiatry.

Many of you will follow this same kind of path in making your final choice, finding two or three specialties that appeal to you and then weighing the advantages and disadvantages of each. The important thing is to have all the information you can so that your decision is informed and intelligent.

But if, even after all this effort, you have difficulty making a choice, you can apply for a transitional year program. Say, for example, that you have narrowed your choice to a medicine or a surgical subspecialty. You can take a PGY-1 in general medicine or general surgery to get as much exposure as possible to different subspecialties. Then, for your second year, you apply for the one you finally choose.

After you decide on your specialty, your next problem is selecting the place to do your residency. Again, you need to do a great deal of research before choosing a program. The AMA publishes a directory of training programs, usually in the spring. Many specialties publish their own directories with more detailed information. AMSA puts out the *Student Guide to the Appraisal and Selection of House Staff Training Programs.* Also, your counselor or advisor can help you find a program suited to you. He or she will probably know people in programs around the country.

One place to begin is by choosing a geographic area you like. For some of you, this will not be an important consideration. But remember that eighty percent of the physicians finishing residency stay in the area where they did their residency. If you know that you'd like to practice in a particular area and setting, urban, suburban, or rural, try to train in that area in a similar setting.

But if you want to train in a major metropolitan area or in a small community hospital, for example, be sure to see what the future of the program looks like. After you finish residency, "Where did you train?" is a question you will be asked repeatedly. Much of your professional network is based on the people in your training program. Some programs that are not university affiliated are in trouble because of funding problems. But if physicians there are heavily involved in research, they're most likely bringing in grant money to support the research—and, as a result, the program.

You also will have to choose between a university-hospital or a community-hospital program. If you want to go into research or academic medicine, a university-based program will provide more opportunity to work with people doing research and to do it yourself. A university-based program will also help you develop a network among medical academicians. A professor at a well known medical school said that he could not think of one attending in a major teaching program who did not come out of a university-based program.

Once you have narrowed the possibilities, talk to as many people, both physicians and residents, as you can who are working in the programs. This kind of first-hand information is important, for one reason because the programs change so rapidly. People at Harvard Medical School, in fact, think this information is so important that each year they send a questionnaire to residents in every program in the country asking for information about the program and for their impressions of it.

Some of you may wish to consider the Armed Services Residency Program. If you are interested in aerospace medicine, you should definitely look into this program because most of the residencies in aerospace medicine are offered through the Air Force. To be accepted for a military residency, you must qualify for commission in one of the branches of the armed services. Because these residencies are highly competitive, you need to begin planning early—at least by your second year of medical school. For more information about the programs, go to the local recruiting offices of the three branches.

After deciding where you want to go, you need to send in applications. Remember that applications and your curriculum vitae (CV) should be typed, be complete, be accurate, and be neat. As one physician who screens applicants said, "If they leave out information on something as important as this, what are they going to do with histories? Besides, I don't like what it says about their attention to detail." In talking about how sloppy some applications are, another said, "We need to give the appearance of being neat, even if we aren't. Sloppy applications suggest sloppy work." Anything you have to write for the application should also be neat and correct, with no grammar or punctuation errors. Again, physicians have no room for even small errors. And errors in your writing may mean to some of the people reading it that you are not concerned about minor errors.

You will also need to supply references. And, even if you are an AMG at the top of your class in the most prestigious medical school in the country, one bad letter of reference or one poor informal phone reference check will seriously harm your chances of getting into a good program. Although your references are asked about your clinical expertise, most of the questions are about your interpersonal skills—something else you need to begin working on early in medical school. (See Chapter III, "Building Your Network.")

Your next step is to schedule interviews. Try to do this as early as you can, before some of the more competitive programs have no more interview slots left in the schedule. Also try to plan your rotations practically so you have time to interview.

Before you go for an interview, find out *everything* you possibly can about the program and about the people who will be interviewing you, especially the chairperson. One famous chairperson, for example, asks all applicants if they smoke. In more than twenty years, he has not accepted *one* person who said yes. However, at least one person, who had done his homework, answered no and then spent his residency hiding his smoking. Ten years later the chairperson still does not know he smokes.

Be sure to try to interview with the chairpeople of the programs, to see how you interact with them. As you finish residency, they are the ones who will identify most of the jobs for you. They also will serve as your primary professional reference. If you find a chairperson with whom you have no rapport now, there is not much chance that you will have in four or five years. So you might be better off considering another program.

If you are nervous about interviewing, check with your student affairs office to see if it offers help. Some schools do videotapes of mock interviews; others do dry runs. If the school does not have anything, role-play with other students. Also, Chapter VIII, "Surviving the Interview Process," although meant for people coming out of residency, has some general advice on interviewing. Perhaps the most important thing for you to remember is the advice of the director of a resident training program in the Northwest: "Remember the famous commercial: Never let them see you sweat. Doctors have to be cool—no matter how tense the situation."

Throughout the process of applying and interviewing, be sure to keep copies of everything you send and to get the names—correctly—of all the people you talk to, both in person and on the phone. An easy and efficient way to keep track of people you talk to in person is to get their business cards. You can even buy a business-card file to keep them in. Make notes about what you discuss in your interviews and in important phone calls. Then, when it comes time to sign up for the Match, you'll have before you all the information you need to make your choices.

The Match is essentially just that—a match of hospitals' top choices of applicants with applicants' top choices of hospitals. Most people get their training program through the National Residency Matching Program (NRMP) a private organization. But some specialties and the military have their own matches, all on earlier timetables than the NRMP's. Even if you participate in one of these, you should also sign up for the NRMP match. In the late spring of your third year, you will receive NRMP's agreement form. Sign it, usually sometime in July, and return it with the application fee.

In January of your last year, you send in your ranked list of programs. (You are charged for each one after ten.) The hospitals send in their lists at the same time. One important thing: It is all right to take a chance and list as your number one choice a program you want but think you have little chance of getting. Even if you do not get it, your chances for getting into your second choice are not hurt. Everything is fed into a computer, and on Match Day—usually the second Wednesday in March, even though some people think it should be moved permanently to the Ides of March—you learn your fate.

Some of you, unfortunately, will have learned yours the Monday before Match Day. If you are not matched, that is the day you find out. The reasons for not being matched are usually unrelated to your competency. The director of a resident advising program, a physician, said, "Our residents who aren't matched often applied to only two or three programs or only to top programs in competitive specialties. Maybe one or two a year aren't matched because they have poor clinical skills. Even then, they might do fine in another specialty, but sometimes they don't want to listen when their attendings tell them they're not suited to the specialty they want."

If you do not match, you still have a chance. Some of the positions are not matched either. Your medical school will be notified of the available openings, and at noon EST on the day after Match Day, you can begin phoning hospitals with openings in your specialty. Be prepared. Review your choices with your advisor. Have your CV and transcript in front of you so you can answer questions quickly and accurately. In her chapter "What to Do if You Don't Match," Taylor even suggests that you bring a map so you can see where the hospitals are located and that you bring your spouse or significant other in case you have to decide immediately about an opening that would mean you would have to relocate. She also advises that you have a back-up specialty.

If you feel as if your life is over because you did not get into the program you wanted, you may, once you begin your training, discover that all really is for the best. Many small, community hospital based programs are quite good and offer a breadth of experience that you would not get in a large, major urban program.

Last year, for example, when two surgeon candidates were presented to a community hospital that needed an additional surgeon, the candidate coming out of a large, nationally known program lost out to the one from a small, community hospital based program. The candidate from the smaller program had a wider range of experience in performing surgery in some of the more specific subspecialty areas, often as the primary surgeon. The candidate from the larger program had been limited to general surgery because the physicians in the subspecialties performed the surgery in those areas.

Perhaps the best advice comes from the orthopedic resident who is thinking of doing a second residency: "Finally, you should follow your heart. You know in your heart what you want to do, where you'll work best. If you don't follow your heart, you'll always feel the void, the emptiness."

If you know what you want to do, even if it will not bring you as much prestige or money or free time, and if you think realistically that you can do it, even though people think you cannot, try for it. After all, where would we be if Beethoven had listened to his music teacher who told him he had no talent for composition or if Walt Disney had believed the editor who fired him from the newspaper because he did not have good ideas.

Chapter III

Building Your Network

Networking is the basis of your career. It will help you be admitted into a good resident training program, find a good job, and get referrals. You should begin networking from the first day of medical school. What is networking? It is building a personal referral file, getting to know people in all areas of medicine and, later, in your specialty and in your community. But it is more than just having people know you; it is having them like and respect you, as well.

Your residency advisor calls his old friend who is now the department chair of the program you want to get into, your department chair refers you to one of her colleagues, the resident who left two years ago calls to ask if you would like to join his group, your attending gives your name when someone she trained with calls and says, "We're looking for someone to join our group, someone who will fit in and has the same work ethic"—that is networking. How do you think the people in the top programs in your specialty found their great researchers and teachers? Not through ads—through networking.

Networking is the best possible way to find a job, primarily because you have no competition. You can respond to ads and mass market yourself forever, but nothing beats a personal referral. As one San Francisco physician who is involved in a search for his large multi-specialty group said, "After the first two, all those CVs and transcripts and letters look alike." How does he sort out the applications? "If I see a name I know or the person comes from a program where I know somebody, I give them a call."

There is a paradox, though. The old saying "It's not what you know but who you know" does not always apply in medicine. To get into a residency program, to get a job, to get referrals, you have to have good grades and board scores, and you have to be clinically competent. If you do not have good grades and board scores, if you are not an excellent clinician, you can be the nicest person around, but you will not get into a good program or get a good job. Technical knowledge and expertise are expected. One chairperson of medicine said, "I look first for very good credentials. I can tell about eighty percent from a person's CV—but many people have very good credentials."

That is the problem. Almost every one of you is clinically competent; if you were not, you would not be where you are now. At one well known university, a ninety-three or ninety-four on a test in a famous science course is a C. Most of you got As and Bs. So how do people make choices among you? Usually by asking people they know what the people can tell them about you, about your personality. The same chairperson said, "I always try to find a contact at the referring institution."

In addition to the fact that most of you are good, if not excellent, clinicians, the increased competition at all levels of medicine makes choosing among you difficult. So the days of being able to survive on your technical skills alone are gone. You need good people skills as well. Physicians who are brusque with patients, irritable with nurses and ancillary staff, and antagonistic to administrators will find themselves being passed over for jobs. People hire people they like.

Many of you are working so hard in your residency at improving your technical, or "hard," skills that you tend to forget about developing your "soft" skills. The chief of a physical medicine and rehabilitation department has said, "Some residents seem to have tunnel vision. They forget along the way how important the people they're working with—at all levels—will be to them."

One reason that your soft skills have become so important is the "incorporation" of medicine. Almost all of you will be working for, or at least with, other people. And one of the things that happens in the corporate world is that people hire people in their own image. One Fortune 100 company, for example, has a strong corporate culture and personality. Through elaborate testing and interviewing of prospective employees, the company weeds out people who do not fit. They might have A's in their courses, but unless the company needs their skills *and* can bury them in research, they will not be hired.

One physician said that choosing a partner or a group member is "more difficult than choosing a wife. You spend more time together and often work more closely. The economic and, more important, the philosophic success of the partnership or group depends on a good fit."

When asked what he looked for while interviewing for a fourth member of his group, an otolaryngologist said, "A good person— someone who has moral integrity, is not out to make a bundle, and wants to develop good patient relationships. You have to realize that by the time these people get through training, they know what they have to know. They all have four fingers and a thumb; they don't have five thumbs. We're looking for other things....

"We want to know what their priorities are. Are they interested in building a practice? Or are they just interested in how much time off they'll have or how much money they'll get? We don't want fat egos. We had one guy here who thought he was God's gift to medicine— cool, calculating, egotistical. We didn't even give him another look. We bring back the people who want to know what they can do for themselves rather than what they'll be given."

In addition to having your corporate fit judged by other physicians, you will often be judged by hospital or health-care corporation administrators and lay board members. These people have traditionally been the physician's antagonists, but in the new world of survival through cooperation, they will often be part of the interviewing team. One CEO of a large, for-profit joint venture said about a job candidate, "He was excellent—highly skilled, out of one of the best programs in the country. Unfortunately, when we went out together for a walk on the water, I drowned. We can't really use people like that here. We need people who can work well with everyone."

You have to remember that the *real* information about you is discovered in telephone reference checks, not in letters. You need letters because they are important for credentialing, but people do not like to commit themselves in writing. Letters are too open to deposition. For example, the attending who said on the telephone, "He's an excellent doctor. But I'd never work with the s.o.b.," said in his letter of reference: "Dr. Doe is an excellent clinician." It was the telephone call that turned up the bad news.

Also, many letters of reference are not written by the person signing them. They may be form letters. Or they may have been written by a secretary for the person's signature. Sometimes they are even written by the job candidates themselves. As a result, people hiring seldom, if ever, rely solely on letters.

The chairman of medicine said, "Letters *never* have negatives. When I see a flat letter, one that's good but with no superlatives, or when I get a general letter of reference, I always make a point of phoning someone whom I know and who knows the candidate to dig for more information. The only letter I pay close attention to is the one that says, 'I'd like so-and-so to stay....Your program would be fortunate to attract a physician of this caliber.' That letter's an open door."

In an editorial in the Ohio State newsletter, Ernie Johnson, chairperson of physical medicine and rehabilitation at Ohio State, advises search committees to "confirm references with phone calls!" He then lists some "code words" in letters of reference:

"superb clinician"—illiterate

"aggressive"—requires disrobing for a curbstone consult

"fine one-on-one teacher"—20 "y'knows" and 15 "ahs" per 15 minutes of lecture

"well-funded researcher"—travels the old-boy circuit but can't take a blood pressure. Never has drawn blood and needs an operating manual to get the "Ankle Jerk."

He also says, "We need...critical and reliable information from friends and faculty colleagues,...to separate the sheep from the goats." That information comes from phone calls.

What specifically are your references asked? (See Figure 2 for an example of a reference check sheet.)

HOW DO YOU RELATE TO PATIENTS?

The attending said of the s.o.b. OB/GYN, "He talks down to patients in the clinic. He berates the young, expectant mothers from low socioeconomic groups and treats them like dirt. He's very controlling. In fact, I think he hates women."

In his interviews with prospective physicians, a chairman of an

REFERENCE CHECKS   Reference's name _____

Candidate: _____   Address _____
Date & Time: _____   _____
Recruiter: _____ Phone # _____ (Home) _____ (Office) _____
  1. How long have you known Dr. _____? _____ years.
  2. Would you send your family to Dr. _____ for care?
  3. On a scale of 1 to 10, how would you compare Dr. _____
     to others (on the current level)? _____
  4. Managerial abilities _____
  5. Clinical judgment (technical ability) _____
  6. Rapport with patients _____
  7. Compatibility with colleagues _____
  8. Ability in speaking and writing English _____
  9. Personal appearance _____
 10. Flexibility in adjusting to new ideas and techniques _____
 11. How does the doctor relate to support personnel? _____
 12. Work habits_____
 13. Willingness to work (workaholic vs. lazy)_____
 14. To your knowledge, are there any malpractice suits pending? __
     _____
 15. Any indications of chemical dependency? _____
 16. What is the doctor's strongest asset? _____
     _____
 17. What are the areas in which the doctor could improve? _____
     _____
 18. Anything else that you feel a colleague should be aware of con-
     cerning Dr. _____ or his/her family? _____
     _____
 19. Do you think Dr. _____would do well in this position?
 20. Would you hire Dr. _____? _____

Source: Garofalo, Curtiss & Company, Ardmore, Pennsylvania.

Figure 2

OB/GYN department in Texas assesses their attitude toward patients by asking, "Who delivers the baby?" If they answer, "I do" or "The doctor does," they do not get the job. Why? "The mother delivers the baby. We're just there to help out."

Very often in residency you work with patients you do not like. One physician said that because many of her indigent clinic patients were not people she would "like to know," she just thought of them by diagnosis and room number, not by name—the gall bladder in 204. She really believed that her interpersonal skills with these patients were excellent and could not understand the concern of her chairperson and attendings.

Another resident in a large urban program described how she tries to deal with the problem: "I can't deny that I get very irritated and impatient. These people come in and I never know what's going on with them. They may come in weeks after they were supposed to. They probably didn't take their medication, and if they did, they probably took it erratically. The list goes on and on. I just keep trying to remind myself that I chose medicine because I want to help people. And these people sure need help. I keep trying to find the person in there."

Surprisingly, another difficult patient is the Yuppie. Yuppies are accustomed to being assertive and to asking questions and to insisting on their rights. You may have to spend more time than you want or think you should explaining procedures, drawing pictures, and justifying what you are doing.

But no matter how difficult the patient, you cannot afford to be condescending or cold or brusque. You have to "keep trying to find the person in there."

HOW DO YOU RELATE TO YOUR CHAIRPERSON AND ATTENDINGS?

This question is probably the most crucial because these are the people who will most likely be your references.

On grand rounds do you bluff your way through or hide in the back of the crowd? Remember that in residency you are not expected to be omniscient; you are there to learn. So do not be afraid to admit you do not know something. Before grand rounds, for example, one resident studies the cases and tries to determine the questions she might be asked. When she comes to one she does not know, she asks the question before someone can ask her. Instead of seeing her as a dimwit, her attendings see her as thoughtful, insightful, and prepared.

When you do make a mistake, do you admit you did? Again, you are not expected to be perfect. Everyone occasionally makes misdiagnoses or performs a procedure incorrectly. When you do, own up to it. Being able to say to an attending, "I was wrong," is very important. You need to be able to recognize your weaknesses. If you do not, you will be seen as insecure and dishonest.

How well do you take directions? Do you get them right the first time and follow through with what you are asked to do? Early in your residency especially you will be given many directions. And your attendings are not going to expect much questioning of what you are asked to do. Back to the s.o.b. OB/GYN: "Every time he was asked to do something, he always had some new idea. He kept pushing every new technique and idea before they had been thoroughly tested. He really believed he knew more than the rest of us. I think the only reason he could find for being in training and not practicing without a license was fear of prison."

If you do have questions about something you are asked to do, at least be tactful when you ask them. Do not be arrogant and constantly challenge the authority of your chairperson and attendings. One of the ways they are judging you is on your willingness to learn and change. In a telephone interview, one attending said of a cardiology resident, "She always insists that her way is best. She doesn't listen to what we say or seem to think we have anything to teach her. She doesn't realize that anything as complex as medicine is going to be changing all the time. I'd want someone a little more flexible working with me, someone who's not so rigid."

HOW WELL DO YOU RELATE TO STAFF?

Do not be arrogant to your ancillary staff either. Some of them may, in fact, be asked about you. Having tantrums when they do not do things your way, throwing instrument trays on the floor when they are not made up to suit you, brushing aside the professional advice of your staff—none of these do much toward building your network. They may, in fact, result in your being disciplined or even dismissed. Because of the nursing shortage, nurses have become a real power in hospitals.

The ICU nurse with 15 years of experience may know more about a procedure than you do. Listen to what she has to say; be willing to ask her advice. Treating the staff like idiots will not make you seem to be a great physician. As one long-time nurse said, "I've worked with lots of residents. And what I've found is that the most difficult ones are usually the most insecure. The good ones aren't afraid to ask me what I would do or what I think about something. I almost feel sorry for the others. I'm a mother, and I want to take them aside and say, 'Look, it's okay to act as though I know something you don't. Nobody's going to think you're stupid.'"

When a patient went into a small beach emergency room to have a fishhook removed from her finger, the resident on duty, referring to himself as "we," began a lengthy discourse on his "preferred method of treatment." After a while, the middle-aged nurse said, "Excuse me, doctor, but would you like me to cut off the rest of the tackle?"—another hook, a sinker, and about a yard of leader that had been dangling from the patient's finger as the resident talked. After waiting a few seconds to impress upon the nurse her impertinence, he answered, "Of course!" The nurses smiled at each other. The patient interrupted to tell him just to shove the hook through and cut off the barb. And she went back to the beach to regale her neighbors with an imitation of the "nervous ten-year-old pretending to be a doctor."

You also need to be willing to help with scut work. Standing back from work you consider beneath your dignity when that work clearly needs to be done and everyone else is too busy will not make you seem more important. It will probably make you seem unemployable. Remember the team player.

Another consideration in your relationship with the staff is how well you handle your authority with them, how well you are able to elicit their cooperation. Barking out orders and insisting on deference, being stern and unbending will not make you seem like a better doctor and certainly will not command respect. Respect is earned, not given.

One resident, when asked what he considered his greatest strength, answered, "Getting people to do what I want." How? "By relying a lot on people's intelligence and training and experience." When therapists, for example, ask him what treatment he suggests, he asks what they have in mind. If their treatment is different from the one he wants, he praises their ideas and then asks if they had considered the treatment he wants. Usually they "rush off to do exactly what I want." Manipulative? Perhaps. But this way, everybody wins—including the patient.

HOW WELL DO YOU RELATE TO YOUR PEERS?

When asked what his relationship with his fellow residents was like, one physician answered, "Well, it's okay." When the interviewer said, "Tell me about 'okay,'" he said, "Well, I hate to sound egotistical. It's just that I honestly believe that intellectually I'm far ahead of them. As a result, I tend to work more with attendings. I don't spend much time with the other residents." In a phone reference check, one of those attendings said, "Dr. [Smith] is by far the brightest resident in our program. But instead of sharing what he knows—you know, helping the others along—he tends to ignore them....I don't think he'd work too well with other people."

Given the competitive nature of medical education (remember the people who trashed your experiments in biology lab), medical students often put so much effort into trying to impress the people making decisions about them that they tend to forget about their peers. An assistant dean of a medical school has called medical education an *infantilizing process:* "[Medical students] probably more than any others spend most of their educational lives working under strong authority figures—you know, the old God syndrome. Some of them can't see anything but 'How can I please Daddy?' They're like those little cherubs on the playground who smile beatifically at the parents and then bash the other kids over the head with their sandbuckets."

Do not get so caught up in your own career track that you forget about the people racing along beside you. Share your information with them. Your chairperson and attendings will still know you are bright.

Pick up on the signals people around you are sending out. After all, physicians are expected to be acutely sensitive. When you see one of your peers suffering from sleep deprivation, offer to help out. Be there for your peers. When you leave training, peers are all you will have.

Dr. Smith's chances in the job market would have been much better had the attending said of him, "Dr. Smith is one of the brightest residents we have. And he's always willing to help out people who don't know quite as much or who have a harder time learning." Over and over again prospective employers say that they are looking for team players, that they do not want cutthroats with bloated egos. If your references say that you ignore your peers or, worse, that you see them floundering and let them sink, why should employers think you will act differently with them when they become your peers?

WHAT IS YOUR APPEARANCE LIKE?

The modern physician is expected to be well groomed and to dress professionally. A recent survey published in the *Journal of the American Medical Association* (JAMA) turned up the following facts. Sixty-five percent of the two hundred patients interviewed want their physicians in white coats; fifty-two percent say no jeans; thirty-seven percent want their male physicians to wear ties; thirty-four percent want their female physicians to wear skirts.

One eighty-year-old dowager in a famous West Coast clinic told the resident coming in to do a preop procedure, "Young man, don't even think of coming near me. Your shirt is crumpled, your nails are dirty and ragged, and you need a haircut. Send in someone who looks like a doctor. *You* look like an aging hippy."

HOW WELL DO YOU SPEAK AND WRITE?

In the busy and often chaotic world of medicine, physicians have to communicate clearly and directly. Instructions, either written or verbal, that have to be decoded waste too much time. And they are potentially dangerous. At one East Coast hospital a surgeon performed a double radical mastectomy on a woman who had only benign cysts. Why? He misunderstood the pathologist's report.

Establishing good patient relationships involves explaining often complicated diagnoses and treatments as simply and effectively as you can. Who would ever trust his or her life to the physician who, instead of saying a patient died, said the patient "failed to fulfill his wellness potential"?

ARE YOU PUNCTUAL?

One chairperson said, "The best residents wear high speed shoes." Chronic lateness, besides suggesting a psychological problem, creates havoc with scheduling. Your performing a seven a.m. procedure at seven thirty-five throws off the entire day.

Long waits infuriate patients, something you cannot afford to do in the scramble for patients. One patient called her physician of twenty years to renew her seizure medicine, but he told her she would have to come in for a checkup, even though she had a physical scheduled for the following week. A busy professional herself, she scheduled the earliest appointment, arrived on time, and waited for an hour before the physician even arrived at the office. Once there, "he waltzed around the office swinging his coffee cup and chatting and laughing with his staff. When I was finally called in—one and a half hours late—he made no apology at all for being late."

He took her blood pressure, asked her how she was, and gave her the prescription—no EEG then, nor was one scheduled for the following week. "I asked him why, if all he was going to do was take my blood pressure, he couldn't have just phoned in the prescription. He said, 'Physicians don't diagnose over the phone.' He got my thirty dollars, but he lost a patient—five if you count my family. We never went near him again, and I tell everyone I can to avoid him."

Potential employers are particularly concerned about punctuality. One person's being late can disrupt an entire office. Also, being late with your charting holds up reimbursement—and being really late might even mean you will not get it.

HOW WELL DO YOU DO YOUR CHARTING AND PAPERWORK?

Your charting and paperwork are signs of how you treat your job. If you do not take responsibility for doing them, you are probably seen as generally not very responsible. If you are careless with them, you are probably seen as generally careless. No one likes to do charting. But it does have to be done, and it has to be done accurately and punctually.

Not filling out the correct forms accurately and not sending them in on time can cost you and your employers a great deal of money because you will not be reimbursed. If your colleagues do not like you, whether you are a resident or an attending, charting is where they can get you. They can document your errors and then use them to discipline you—perhaps put a note in your file or suspend your admitting privileges. One multispecialty group, for example, is firing a general surgeon because he is so careless about his paperwork and so late getting in the forms that he constantly disrupts the group's cash flow. Then there are the times when he does not collect at all because of error or lateness.

Also, with malpractice hanging over your shoulder every time you see a patient, you cannot afford to make mistakes or to leave out important information when you do your paperwork. Those mistakes and careless omissions are the things that lawsuits are made of.

WHAT IS YOUR GENERAL ATTITUDE?

Most of you spend most of your time worn out from your demanding schedules. When you are exhausted, being polite and paying attention are difficult. But if you want to be seen as someone who is warm, caring, tactful—a team player—you will have to force yourself to focus positively on patients and staff, no matter how tired you are.

One way to stay alert to the people around you even when you think you cannot is to practice reflective listening. If, even after listening carefully, you are not sure you understand what someone says, paraphrase the statement. When, for example, you do not know whether the nurse is concerned about Mrs. Smith's EKG results or is just reporting them to you, ask, "Did I understand you to say that you're concerned about Mrs. Smith's EKG?" The nurse can then clarify what she meant. And you have accomplished two things: you have made the nurse feel that you care about her opinions, and you have elicited information that will enable you to respond intelligently rather than vaguely.

You can use the same technique with your attendings. Using reflective listening forces them to clarify what they have asked, gives you time to think of the answer, and makes you appear interested and eager to learn. Using it with your patients makes them feel that you are genuinely interested in their concerns.

Other qualities that are being assessed under this general question are things such as loyalty, trustworthiness, and honesty. Now that most physicians work with other people rather than by themselves, these traits have taken on increased importance.

DO YOU HAVE ANY CHEMICAL DEPENDENCIES?

Obviously, if you do have a dependency now, your employment picture is not bright. But if you did have one and you have been through rehabilitation or have effected your own cure, do not lie. Somehow the people hiring will always find out. When they do, they have to cope not only with your problem but also with your lying.

One very bright young physician had been through rehabilitation and had been clean for two years. When he asked his chairperson what he should say about the problem, the chairperson said he did not think it was important anymore so not to mention it and to say "no" on the licensing application.

Because both his technical and interpersonal skills were excellent, the physician found a job in a six-physician group in Colorado—the place he wanted to be because he is a skier. Six months after he started the job, his engagement ended bitterly. His ex-fiancée, another physician, called his employers and told them about his dependency. They had to fire him, primarily because he had lied to them. When asked if they would have hired him if they had known, they said probably not. But they were not sure if their judgment was skewed now by his lying.

The next time around he told the truth, was hired, and is now successfully, and happily, practicing medicine. This time he is in Utah, which he thinks has even better skiing.

Your references are usually asked two open-ended questions: Would you hire this physician? Would you send a member of your family to this physician? These are usually the questions that reveal the most about you. Someone who does not really want to recommend you but also does not want to ruin your chances can answer most of the other questions fairly neutrally. It is here that the people checking your references listen for pauses, for hesitations and then move in.

One way to try to see yourself is to ask yourself the same questions and to try to answer them as objectively as possible. *Would you hire yourself or send a member of your family to someone like you?* How would you answer the question "What will your references say about you?"

If, when you try to answer the question, you do not like what you see about yourself, if you think your soft skills are in pretty bad shape, you can still do something about building your network. You can begin to change so that when your chairperson or your attendings are asked about you, they will say, "Dr. Smith used to be abrupt and egotistical, but lately we've seen real improvement." In trying to change your image, you are not being manipulative or dishonest. You are actually displaying a capacity for growth, something that all employers value highly.

What if you are going through a bad time right now—a divorce, perhaps, and you have been irritable and short tempered? Most people have been through bad times themselves and will understand that your current behavior is an aberration, if you let people know what is happening to you. Again, do not try to be perfect. Apologize when you act out of character. Not explaining your actions may make people think that you have become puffed up with your own consequence and position. Although you cannot use personal problems as an excuse forever, telling the people you work with will make them sympathetic rather than critical.

What happens if you have a genuine personality conflict with one of your attendings, and you know he or she will give you a bad reference. One bad reference is not the end of the world. The people checking your references will ask many people about you to try to build up a picture of you. If they get a bad reference, they put it into context. The problem comes when the picture is of an aloof, self-centered, rude know-it-all.

One chairperson has said that in medical training "We first must develop competence. Only with competence can we develop confidence. And only with confidence can we develop compassion. We ask too much if we look for that real compassion that makes a great doctor before the third year of residency." So you do have time to develop your people skills. The important thing is that you develop them. Without them, your medical career will be circumscribed and unfulfilling. As the chairperson of medicine said, "Modern medicine doesn't really have room for the high friction individual."

You might do well to remember Emily Dickinson's poem:

> Surgeons must be very careful
> When they take the knife.
> Underneath their fine incisions
> Stirs the culprit, life.

No matter how fine your incisions, how you deal with the culprit life—with its difficult patients, charts and paperwork, exhausting schedules, demanding colleagues—is what you will be judged on.

Chapter IV

Assessing Your Needs

Before you look for a job, you have to determine what you want. Not what you want for a job—what you *want:* what you need to make your life fulfilling. Do you want good bike trails? Do you want to be surrounded by other people in your specialty? Do you want to pay off your debts in two or three years? You may want all of these, and perhaps you will be lucky and find them all in one place. Most of you, though, will have to make trade-offs. But before you begin making trade-offs, you have to decide those things that you cannot trade off, those things that are essential to you.

If you are going to be happy in your job, you have to look carefully at who you are. Just as you did when you chose your residency, you must determine what is important to you. Do not think that important things will not matter. Or you may end up like the physician who, against good advice, took a job in a small town in West Virginia. He was an Orthodox Jew who strictly adhered to the dietary laws. Most of the people in the town did not even know what kosher meant. After eating tuna fish for nine months, with occasional weekend splurges in Washington, D.C., he called the person who had helped him find the job and said, "Get me out. I hate tuna fish. And you were right—I should never have come here." He now practices in a large Mid-Atlantic urban area.

Even though you have some things that you absolutely cannot trade off, you have to be flexible. In choosing your first job, set short-term rather than long-term goals and try to fit your short-term into your long-term goals. Physicians average two to three job changes per career, with the average slightly higher for physicians in academic medicine. Once you have determined your ideal position, think of the steps you will have to take to get it.

And think of those steps in three- to five-year blocks. A child psychiatrist, for example, knows that eventually she wants to build her own child and adolescent psychiatry facility in New England. For her first job, she accepted a position with a hospital in the Southwest, a place where she does not particularly want to live. But because she is starting up a new child and adolescent psychiatry unit there, she took the job to get the administrative experience she will need when she has her own facility.

Even if you are not sure of your long-term goals, you can determine what would satisfy your needs for the next five years or so. Perhaps you are like the ophthalmologist who was not really sure where he wanted to practice or what kind of practice model he wanted to be in. But he did know that he wanted to pay off his almost six-figure debt and that he wanted his wife to be able to stay home with their three young children. So he decided to take a job where he could make *lots* of money. A hospital in northern North Dakota brought him in and set up his office.

One Christmas day, when he was on call and his wife and children had gone home to visit her parents in California, he was standing in his kitchen talking on the telephone—wearing his hat and coat. When the caller asked why, he answered, "It's forty below zero. I've never been so cold in my life." And after a pause, "I've never had this much money either." In four years, he cleared his debts and took a job in southern California. But for those four years, because he knew what he wanted, he was able to live happily in an environment that he did not like.

For some of you, achieving your long-term goals might mean opting for additional training rather than for a job. You might have decided to do a second residency. Like the resident in orthopedics, you may have decided to follow your head rather than to "follow your heart" in choosing your residency. But you have discovered by now that you would be much happier in the field that you originally rejected "for practical reasons." Or during residency you may have become interested in one of your field's subspecialties, and you have decided to take a fellowship in that area.

Some of you decide to continue training because you are waiting for spouses or significant others to finish their education or training. So rather than sign on at a large group or HMO for a year or so, you might take a fellowship. Continued training is also a way of buying time until you determine what you want to do.

Some of you decide to continue training because you want to put off entering the "real" world, because you find the thought of leaving too unsettling. When asked what he was going to do for a job next year, a chief resident of medicine smiled and said, "I'm taking a fellowship next year." Why? "We get used to this environment; we're protected here. And everything's black and white. Medical education doesn't prepare you for gray, only for black and white. If I'm sitting in an office next year and you come in with a pain in your chest, you could have a hundred things wrong with you. I'm not ready to deal with a hundred possibilities."

Whatever your reasons for choosing continued training over a job, doing another residency or a fellowship has definite advantages. Perhaps the most important is that when you do go out to find a job, you will probably have more cards to play with. Getting the job you want may be much easier.

The great disadvantage of continued training is the relatively low salary you get in residency or in a fellowship program. Another disadvantage is that although continued training may give you an initial edge, in a few years rapidly changing technology may make the skills and procedures you learn for your subspecialty obsolete. In the long run, a broader-based training may be more practical.

Besides continued training, another choice for those of you not yet ready to move into practice is to be a locum tenens. Locum tenens are "temps" hired daily, weekly, or monthly to provide patient care in the absence of the regular physician. You might be filling in during vacations, protracted illnesses, or job searches. Reimbursement varies according to specialty and geographic area. The advantage of being a locum is that you are able to practice in a variety of practice modes and settings. Also, you do not have to tie yourself to one job for two or three years.

For those of you ready to move into practice, you will probably base your choice on three things: your lifestyle needs, your professional needs, and your financial needs.

LIFESTYLE NEEDS

Unless you have very strong professional or financial needs—you want to be in an academic environment or you have a six-figure debt—

being able to live the lifestyle you want in the place you want to live it will often be the determining factor in your choice of a job. Discounting your personal needs would be a great error, unless you do not mind eating tuna fish every day.

One physician went to look at a job in the mountains. Professionally and financially, she found it to be everything she wanted. But she turned it down. When asked why, she answered, "Besides medicine, two things in my life are very important to me, astronomy and jogging. There's so much fog out there at night that I'd never be able to see the stars. And I'd kill myself trying to run. The only places to run are up mountain roads or down them. I'd never be happy there."

Another physician interviewed for a job that seemed perfect for both him and his wife. Because he plays the violin and has "to be able to hear great music," they wanted to be close to a major orchestra. Because his wife is a weaver and spins and dyes wool from her own sheep, they wanted to be in a place where they could have a small farm. Besides being an excellent professional opportunity, this job provided both proximity to an orchestra and a farm. When he turned down the job, everyone was surprised. But he turned it down because he and his wife are cyclists and the area had no clearly defined bicycle paths.

Although you may be more flexible than these physicians, you should consider a number of things before making your decision. Among them is geography. What kind of climate do you want to live in? Some of you may think that the ophthalmologist in North Dakota was in a northern Eden with snow, skiing, fishing, hunting. Others shudder at the thought of icy weather. You may not be able to live in areas of high humidity. A physician who is in a wheelchair, for example, had to turn down a job in Alabama because the humidity made maneuvering the chair too difficult. Or you may know that extremely hot weather makes you lethargic and irritable. One physician had as her top priority a "cool, dry climate" because she said, "I spent a summer working in a clinic in Louisiana and discovered that hot, humid weather turns me into a monster. I loved the work, but my personal life was shot. I run, and even when I'd run at five-thirty in the morning, I'd end up standing in a giant puddle of sweat."

Do you want to be near mountains or beaches? For many of you the answer to this question will be based on private needs rather than on recreational interests. People usually feel most comfortable in an area similar to the one they grew up in. If you grew up on the plains, the mountains probably make you feel hemmed in, trapped. If you grew up in the mountains, the plains probably make you feel exposed, unprotected.

A general surgeon who had taken a job in northern Vermont has moved to the coast of North Carolina because she grew up ten miles from the ocean. "I never really understood how important having the ocean nearby is to me. I loved Vermont, my colleagues, my patients. But for some reason, I never felt completely at ease there. I didn't realize why until one day when I drove into New Hampshire and felt this great release, as if the world had opened out for me. Suddenly it occurred to me: New Hampshire has an outlet to the sea."

You should also consider the size and type of community you will be most comfortable in. If you, like the writer Fran Liebowitz, think that the outdoors is what you go through to get from your apartment to a taxi and if hunting to you means bargains, you obviously should not even think about a job in a rural, farming area. On the other hand, if you think cities are not even "nice places to visit," stay away from jobs in large metropolitan areas.

Again, the type of community you choose will be determined in large part by the type you grew up in or where you trained. (Remember the eighty percent of you who stay in the area where you train.) One internist left a small city on the edge of megalopolis to take an offer in Los Angeles to be chairman of a large, prestigious department. He and his wife had both grown up in small European cities and had spent the first five years of their marriage in the African jungle. They lasted one year before returning to the small city they had left. Why? "Ze freeways!"

You may decide on the reverse of the kind of place you grew up in. You may have grown up in the city but want a safer, more communal environment for your family. Or you may have grown up in a rural area but want more cultural opportunities for your family. A Hispanic physician who grew up in the WASP, affluent suburb of an East Coast city very carefully chose to practice in an area where his children would be surrounded by other Hispanics. "I felt a terrible sense of isolation when I was growing up. I was different, my parents were different, our food was different. I became shy and introverted. Even in medical school, one of my professors asked me why I didn't contribute more in discussions since I knew so much. My parents thought they were doing the best for us. But I'd never want that for my children."

When deciding on the type of community you want, consider commuting time. How much time will you have to spend in the car? Under what conditions? One physician, a brilliant diagnostician who has also published many highly respected articles in her field, repeatedly turns down offers for "better opportunities." "I *hate* to drive. Here, I live two blocks from my office, so most of the time I walk to work. The hospital is an easy fifteen-minute drive. The tennis club is five minutes away. Why should I leave?"

A major consideration for many of you is social climate. If you are a minority physician, do you really want to go to a place where you might be the only minority professional in town or where you might be subjected to either overt or implied prejudice? After three years, a black radiologist, for example, left a small city on the edge of the Mason-Dixon line.

"My family and I were never the victims of outright prejudice. It was more subtle. The people actually didn't mean it. My wife and I were always carefully invited to official things, but nobody ever called us up and asked us over for a spur-of-the-moment cookout. My son and his best friend, who was white, were in the highest reading group in first grade. Because they couldn't keep still or quiet, the teacher separated them. Guess who was put in the lower reading group? It was things like that. That and the isolation—there just weren't that many people like us around."

If you have strong ethnic or religious needs, do not think they will not matter. It is one thing, for example, to say that driving 50 miles each way every week to the synagogue will not be that bad; it is another to do it. You may say that having the children study Greek and go to Sunday school at an Orthodox church is not *that* important, but you may have trouble dealing with the reality. One reason that the internist left Los Angeles was the lack of good religious schools for his children: "We didn't think it would matter as much as it did." Another physician is leaving her job because she and her husband have found that they really cannot do without a strong Ukrainian community, that they depend on it for emotional support.

What about your cultural and recreational needs? If going to art galleries and the theater is vitally important to your emotional well being, why even consider the Upper Peninsula of Michigan? If skiing is your passion, why think about Florida? One resident has listed as his top priority getting a job in one of the five or six cities that have banked bicycle tracks. He is into speed racing, and he does not want to spend his time driving a long distance to a track.

How important are educational opportunities? Because you have spent most of your life in school and in training, you may take the opportunities for granted. But you need to think about how you will feel if you take a job in a place where they are not available. You should think about whether having access to a large medical library or to lectures by the top people in your field is important to you. Would you be content doing your continuing medical education (CME) by going to one or two conferences each year and by reading journals?

Another thing that many of you have not thought much about—mostly because you have not had much of it—is personal time. How much time do you want for yourself and your family? Especially if you are married or are in a long-term, stable relationship, think carefully about this aspect of your job. Remember the high divorce rate among physicians.

A successful neonatologist is the first and only neonatologist in his area. The obstetricians think he is wonderful, but they worry about him because all he does is work. His practice is too large to handle easily by himself, but it is not large enough to support a partner. He is thinking about bringing someone in, though. For his wife, their one-week vacation in Bermuda was the end of the line: He called home twice a day to check on an infant's blood gases because he was not entirely comfortable with his coverage. "I had two choices—get drunk so I wouldn't think about the coverage or call home and check." His wife says, "I put up with things like his never being able to go to the theater with me. He sent me with the doctors' wives' group. But this was our first vacation since our honeymoon five years ago, and I felt as if twelve infants were lying between him and me. We knew when he took this job that he would be very busy because he's the only [neonatologist] around. But I never thought it would be like this."

If you need personal time and if your family life is important to you, do not take a job where you will be the only physician in your field— unless you want to make a lot of money and your family has agreed to live with your busy schedule for a few years until you make it.

Your family's needs are another important consideration, especially if your spouse has a career too. Then you both have to coordinate priorities and think through what you both want. Each of you should draw up a list of "must haves"—both personal and professional. With the list you will be able to see where you mesh and where you might have to make trade-offs. Doing this *before* you begin your job searches will save both of you time and effort—and will help prevent conflicts when you are in the middle of your decision making.

Again, discounting differences in needs and assuming that "things will work out" is a mistake. Your spouse may say that not having access to good sailing will not *really* matter. But once you are both under the pressure of starting new positions, your spouse may become dissatisfied with not having an important outlet for stress. And a dissatisfied or unhappy spouse will obviously affect your own satisfaction and happiness.

Be careful, too, of assuming that a long commute for one or both of you will not affect you. One couple, a physician and an attorney, each found the "perfect" job. Unfortunately, the jobs were three hundred and fifty miles apart. No problem. They would make lots of money, so they could spend time off together, fly up or down for dinner, talk on the phone whenever they wanted.

Of course, the inevitable happened. The physician, taken on to develop the invasive cardiology practice for a large multispecialty group, found herself with little free time. When she was free, her husband was in the middle of researching a big case. "We never saw each other, and when we did, we tried so hard to have everything perfect that things became very artificial. All the little irritations that build up—you know, why is he working again tonight with Susie, why is she always with Joe?—never got resolved. By the time we realized how far we had drifted apart, it was too late. Now we're in the middle of a divorce neither of us ever expected—or wanted. I call him sometimes, and he calls me. The whole thing makes me sad. I wonder if we'd still be together if one of us had taken a not-so-perfect job."

Even if your spouse is not developing a career, you still need to consider his or her needs. And if you find yourselves at a point where you cannot agree, that may be the time to think about how you could resolve the problem by working on short-term goals. "You come here with me now because this job will provide the experience that will give me more options later. I'll go there with you in five years." When a large university-based hospital called a New Hampshire hematologist to offer him a job, he turned it down. His wife, who has an M.B.A., works in Boston. And "the next move is hers."

If you are a parent, you should consider how you will balance parenting with your professional life. Given our culture's socialization of men and women, establishing this balance is particularly difficult for women. Many women feel angry if they have to curtail their careers but guilty if they do not spend as much time as they think they should with their children.

One physician, staying at home with her four young children and becoming more and more resentful of not being able to continue the career she had trained so hard for, found the resolution to her problem on an afternoon television talk show. An actress being interviewed was asked if she didn't feel guilty about choosing her career over her child. She answered that she had not made a choice, that she was an actress *and* a mother. And she said that she did not want her child at eighteen to have to bear the burden of guilt knowing that her mother had given up "her life" for her. "Hearing this," the physician said, "suddenly made everything clear. I realized that I needed to work out an arrangement where I could be both physician and mother. I began working part time at an outpatient clinic. And when my youngest child started school, I started my own practice."

To be satisfied both personally and professionally, many of you will have to make the same sort of arrangements. You may want to be an employee, either full or part time, so you will have some control over your hours and can balance family and career.

If you have children, you also have to think about their needs—and sometimes your needs in terms of what you want for them. For most of you the quality of local schools will be a primary consideration. If the public schools are not good, do you want to assume the financial burden of private schools? Good prep schools are currently running around $5,000 per year, more if your children are in higher grades.

If your children are exceptional—gifted, handicapped, learning disabled—you will obviously need to consider the availability and quality of special educational facilities. For example, a dermatologist whose middle child has spina bifida chose to practice in a city with an excellent pediatric orthopedic and rehabilitation facility, even though it is in an area where he and his wife are not entirely comfortable.

You also have to look at the cultural and recreational opportunities available to the children. Will they be able to participate in good athletic programs? Will they have access to good instruction in the arts? Do you want them to be able to go to the theater, the orchestra, museums? A California physician, perhaps betraying his East Coast roots, said, "I'm looking for a new job because I can't stand this life for my kids. It's so bloody uncultured and provincial. 'London? Where's that?' Nobody's been anywhere. Anyway, out here where do you go? Hawaii? Oklahoma? They may be nice places, but I grew up going to the children's concerts on Saturday afternoons and to museums and even the opera. I hated it sometimes, but it's the old story: now I want my kids to have those experiences."

You may not mind not having safe streets for yourself. But do you want them for your children? Think carefully about the kind of community you want your children to grow up in. One physician left New York City after his adolescent daughter was mugged for the second time. Another left an affluent bedroom suburb—and a thriving practice, which he had built up over six years—because he "didn't like the values they were picking up." The family now lives in a small town in Virginia.

How important to you is having your children live near their grandparents? For some people, proximity to their families is a primary consideration, even if they do not have children. If you grew up in a warm, caring extended family, you may feel lost without that kind of support. The black physician who is now practicing in California is seriously thinking about moving back to his hometown. "I miss the sense of community. Everybody knows everybody. They look out for each other. And I really miss my family. I want my children to know what it's like to have Granny up the street and aunts and uncles and cousins."

Sorting through your lifestyle needs—and those of your family—is often the most difficult part of your decision-making process. You have to consider so many variables. Once you have clarified them, sorting through your professional and financial needs is relatively easy.

PROFESSIONAL NEEDS

For your professional needs one of your first considerations should be what kind of practice model you want to be in. Do you want to be in private practice? Or work in an HMO? Do you want to be involved in a joint venture? Or in a doc-in-a-box? Because the number of possibilities and possible combinations of them is so great, they are discussed in a separate chapter, Chapter V, "Determining Your Type of Practice."

Just as important as type, though, is your role in a group or partnership. Think about whether you would enjoy being part of a large group or even of any group, whether you need to work independently, whether you would mind being a small fish in a big pond or vice versa. One cardiologist set up two interviews in Maine. In one, he would be one of three cardiologists working in a large, state-of-the-art hospital. In the other, he would be the only cardiologist working in a smaller, less well equipped hospital.

He left the first interview thinking that nothing could beat that job. He loved the place, the people, the facilities. In fact, he almost gave his verbal commitment but decided he should at least be polite and go to the second interview. When he finished with the second, he began to realize what being his own boss meant to him. He and his wife spent a weekend going over their priorities and decided to go to the smaller hospital where he could work independently. He wants to be an entrepreneur.

How important is having access to peers and mentors? Many of you enjoy the intellectual stimulation and security of being able to discuss difficult cases with your colleagues. Not having other people around in your specialty may make you feel cut off from what is happening in the field. One reason the ophthalmologist in North Dakota wanted to leave was that he felt isolated, with no one to talk to about the things he was doing.

Others of you are perfectly content to do telephone consultations and to find out what is happening from journals. A neurologist who went to Montana because he likes to hunt and fish says, "I keep up by reading the journals, and I go to a couple of meetings every year. If I want to talk something over, I just call up a couple of people I trained with. They're both in the thick of things. I couldn't stand it— it's too incestuous. I don't want to talk about neurology all the time."

You also should think about what kind of typical daily routine suits you best. If you are a general surgeon, for example, working in a community hospital would most likely provide greater variety. You would be able to do many of the procedures that would be denied you in a major metropolitan teaching hospital. There the subspecialists would do them. However, there you would be able to observe and to assist with more difficult and unusual procedures. In a community hospital, you would be able to do more; in a large teaching hospital, you would be able to see more. You have to decide which is more important to you.

Which are you more interested in, primary or referral care? For some specialties, such as surgery or otolaryngology, this is not a consideration. But for others, such as physiatry or internal medicine, it is. Look at the kind of relationship you want to have with your patients. Obviously, if you want long-term relationships, you should opt for primary care or at least for a combination of primary and referral care.

Negotiating to be chairperson of the Department of General Medicine at a large teaching hospital, a nephrologist insisted on having time for his own primary care practice. "I'm the third generation to practice medicine. I'd never be able to think of myself as a doctor if all I did was administrative work and see referrals in my specialty." After a pause, he said, "I still make house calls. Don't tell anyone. They'd put me away."

How important are the hospital facilities available to you? Do you want the latest equipment? If you are a radiologist, for example, do you think you would not be able to practice well unless you had access to a magnetic resonance imager (MRI)? How much does being in a hospital with a large number and variety of departments mean to you? If you are an obstetrician, for example, you may want a Level Three nursery because you do not want to have to refer out difficult births or to separate the mother from the baby after the birth. Is it important for you to be in a place where the latest and most complicated procedures are being performed, where your colleagues are among the leaders in your field?

You also need to think about the professional opportunities for you in the community. Some specialties, for example, need large catchment areas, the primary and secondary service areas. Neurosurgeons need a catchment of about one hundred thousand people or better. Sometimes a hospital may bring you in when there is an insufficient base to support you, where there is no real growth potential for your specialty. The administrative staff of the hospital may not really care if you leave in a year or two because you will have filled some beds in the meantime. One CEO said, "We use him for a couple of years. He fills beds, brings in some new equipment. He uses us to get experience. No bad feelings." No bad feelings, perhaps—if you understand what you are getting into.

What about the competition in the area? Almost everyone coming out of residency seems to want to go to California. Yet the competition is probably higher in California than it is in any other state. One California doctor, complaining about physicians flooding in, said, "I want to build selective gates on every road into here—they will let in everyone but docs."

Do you want built-in referrals? Or do you think scratch-and-dig practice building would be an adventure? Some of you might enjoy being on your own, developing your practice independently. Others of you may want to spend your time doing procedures or research so want to be sure of your referrals. The important thing is to determine which will be more satisfying.

Do you want the opportunity to do research? Is recognition in your field necessary to you? Again, you should think about whether these are so important that you are willing to trade off other things for them. You will not become a famous researcher if you want to practice in a small town in rural America.

On the other hand, if you want community recognition and respect for yourself as a physician, you should practice in a small town or in a blue-collar community. A young physician practicing in a large city is going back home, to a small southern town. She says, "Back there the doctor is somebody important. Here nobody on the street even knows your name, let alone thinks you're special."

FINANCIAL NEEDS

For some of you, money is going to be a primary factor in deciding where and how to practice. But you have to decide just how important it is. If you want to make a lot of money right now, you will probably have to go to an underserved area. A hospital administrator in New York City was asked why the starting salary she was offering a surgical oncologist was so low. She replied, "We don't need to offer more. Everyone wants to be in a major medical mecca, and we're one of them."

Boston, New York, Washington, D.C., Chicago, San Francisco, Los Angeles—they are among the most expensive places to live in the whole country. Yet their starting salaries for physicians are much lower. And the competition is overpowering. All those "medical meccas" have medical schools and training programs dumping residents into the market. Many physicians, though, still think that being in one of these cities is essential to the good practice of medicine. If you are one of these physicians, be prepared to cut back on your financial expectations.

The irony is that physicians practicing only an hour or two away often make up to one-third more money and live in areas with a lower cost of living. One anesthesiologist loves to dance in crowded discos. It is his way of letting off steam. For its dancing as much as for its medicine, he wanted to be in New York City. But he said, "I looked at the starting salaries and said no way. My debts were too high and so was the cost of living there. Now I'm an hour and a half away in a great place, and I have a great job. I've arranged things so that every Friday night I can go to the Red Parrot or Area. I have the best of both worlds."

When considering your financial needs, you need to set realistic short- and long-term goals. If you take a job that is an excellent professional opportunity but does not pay particularly well, be prepared to cope with financial pressures. Or if you take a job that pays well but is not really what you want, be prepared to cope with the stresses in your professional or personal life. And be sure to talk over your decision thoroughly with your spouse. Remember the physician in North Dakota? One of the reasons that he had such a good experience there was his wife's commitment to the same goal of paying off the debt, fast.

The most important thing to realize in all this assessing is that you *will* have to make trade-offs. You want excellent public schools for your children. Iowa has the highest literacy rate in the country and an excellent public school system. If you grew up on the beach in Florida, do you want to go to Iowa? You want to do research in a university-based hospital with all the latest technological advances. These hospitals are in major metropolitan areas. If you grew up on a ranch in the Rocky Mountains, do you want to live in Los Angeles? You are deeply in debt. You find the perfect job, except for the starting salary. If you *have* to pay bills the day you receive them, do you want to take the job?

A hematologist practicing in New York City said, "I ignored some of the professional reservations I had about this job, anything to get to New York. Now I've gone through the four stages of living here. First, I went to see everything. Second, I began to be selective and went to things I really enjoyed, and I spent some time with friends. Third, I spent more time with friends and went out occasionally. Fourth, I'm staying home with my books and my music and my five locks. I've been mugged once and burglarized four times. Now, I'm too tired, too poor, and too paranoid to go out. I'm looking for another job."

When assessing what you want in terms of lifestyle, professional environment, and money, remember that usually you cannot have everything. Just as there is no perfect physician for a job, there is no perfect job.

Chapter V

Determining Your Type of Practice

As you prepare to enter the job market, you are faced with a bewildering number of options that you must consider. In addition to lifestyle needs, basic professional needs, and financial needs, you must determine the type of practice setting that you want to work in. Life was simpler when a new physician could choose the town in which he or she wanted to practice, hang out a shingle, and wait for the patients to come flocking in—no complicated contracts, no negotiations, no multicopy government forms, just the practice of medicine. In the new alphabet soup world of medicine—HMO, PPO, IPA—trying to determine the practice setting you want may seem overwhelming. Where do you begin?

One place would be to understand the meaning of some of the terms that are tossed around in discussions of practice types. You hear terms such as primary care and capitation all the time, but you may have only vague notions of what they mean.

TYPES OF CARE

The three main types of care are primary, referral, and consultation—or a mixture of the three.

Primary Care

Primary care has come to mean the basic medical care traditionally associated with general practice, with long-term doctor-patient relationships. General practitioners, family medicine specialists, pediatricians, OB/GYNs, and internists provide most of primary care.

In large groups and HMOs the primary care physicians are often called the gatekeepers because they are responsible for deciding whether to refer patients to specialists or what procedures or tests the patients need.

Referral Care

Referral care is the care provided usually by specialists at the request of other physicians. If, for example, during a routine physical a pediatrician discovers leukemia, he or she will most likely refer the patient to a pediatric oncologist. Or if a patient asks a primary physician for the name of a good dermatologist, the primary physician will suggest one or two dermatologists in the community. Because this type of care is often complex and involves seeing patients over an extended time, referral care almost always involves patient management. Many practices, especially highly specialized ones such as surgical subspecialties, are built almost entirely on referrals.

Consultation Care

Consultation care is also care provided at the request of other physicians. But it does not involve patient management. The consultant examines the patient, studies the results of the examination and of any tests, and advises the other physician about the case. Almost no practices are built solely on consultation. Those few that are belong to physicians who after years of successful practice have become acknowledged leaders in their fields.

Mixed Care

Many practices are a combination of the three types of care. For example, pediatric nephrologists provide primary care to their regular patients—immunization, routine physical examinations, treatment of the usual childhood illnesses. They provide referral care to patients with complicated kidney or urinary tract problems. And they may provide consultation care by examining patients of other physicians and giving the physicians advice.

TYPES OF REIMBURSEMENT

Unless you are working on a straight salary, your income will depend primarily upon your reimbursement for the services you provide your patients. Although the settings in which reimbursement is made have become complex, reimbursement divides into only two types—fee-for-service and prepaid. Most physicians' incomes are a combination of the two.

Fee-For-Service

Fee-for-service reimbursement is the traditional form of payment for physicians. It is exactly what it says—a specific fee which the patient or third party pays for a specific service. It is the payment received in solo, partnership, and group traditional practice.

Prepaid

With prepaid, or capitation, reimbursement, health-care providers are paid a monthly fee per patient and a specific amount for a specific procedure. The fee is agreed upon in advance and is usually determined by a third party—an HMO, IPA, or PPO.

So, for example, physicians affiliated with an IPA might receive $12.00 per month per patient enrolled in the IPA. Or they might receive their regular fee minus a predetermined percentage, usually between fifteen to twenty-five percent. Then, if the IPA shows a profit over a certain time, this money is distributed equally among its members.

Combination

Many physicians' incomes are based on mixed reimbursement. Physicians in private practice—either solo or group—may have affiliated with two or three IPAs or PPOs. So they receive fee-for-service reimbursement for their patients not enrolled in those prepaid plans and capitation reimbursement for their patients in the plans.

TYPES OF PRACTICE SETTINGS

Practice settings range from the traditional solo practice through other forms of private practice to staff-model HMOs to corporate medicine. Essentially, though, you will be deciding whether to go into some form of private practice, where you will be self-employed, or to become an employee, where you will receive either a straight salary or a salary with some form of bonus or incentive plan.

Solo Practice

Solo private practice is the traditional method of practicing medicine. In it, single, independent physicians are responsible for their entire practices. They set their own fees for their services, and either their patients or their patients' insurers pay the fees. Almost everyone, however, agrees that this form of practice is becoming less an option for young physicians. As David B. Nash predicts in his interesting and informative book, *Future Practice Alternatives in Medicine*, "...the 'cottage industry' of the solo practitioner will soon be extinct."

One reason is steadily increasing paperwork. To survive financially and to protect their patient bases, most physicians are affiliating with an IPA or a PPO or with a number of them. Many patients are covered under Medicare or Medicaid. To compete with prepaid plans, many traditional insurers such as Blue Cross and Blue Shield are instituting some form of payment plan. With all these payment plans the paperwork for the independent physician becomes so time-consuming that many solo practitioners are finding that they must hire business managers just to keep track of billings.

Another reason is proliferating costs. Malpractice insurance can be both difficult to obtain and prohibitive for the independent physician. Salaries and benefits for office and ancillary staff are rising rapidly. Office space and medical supplies and equipment are becoming more expensive. Now that marketing has become a way of life for health-care providers, many physicians cannot compete for their share of the market because they cannot afford marketing and advertising campaigns. With high start-up costs and an initially slow cash flow as a result of their having to build a patient and referral base and of slow pay from the government, many new physicians have to borrow money to stay afloat. Adding this indebtedness to the indebtedness most of you have from medical school can drive the amount of money you owe well into six figures. Fewer young physicians are willing to assume this kind of debt.

Also, because solo practice is a small business, many physicians are put off by the idea of having to divide their time between being a physician and being a businessperson. Even if you hire a business manager, an office manager, and an accountant and you have an attorney, you are ultimately responsible for what happens to your business. Stories abound of physicians being fleeced by their "trusted" employees. You will have to be involved in hiring—and sometimes firing—employees, in determining salary and benefits for your employees, in overseeing billings and orders for equipment and supplies, in refereeing any office disputes. Your medical education has done little to prepare you for this type of career. If you are not interested in business, at least not right now, you will probably be happier in a setting where you will be able to devote more time to medicine and less to business.

Solo practice certainly has not died out, but it flourishes mainly in underserved areas. So if you want to be a solo practitioner—unless you can buy out a practice, something most new physicians cannot afford—you must accept the fact that you will probably be working in a small town or rural area. One of the drawbacks of this type of setting is the lack of colleagues, especially in your specialty. One of the advantages is that often the community hospital will help you set up your practice, will pay your start-up costs, and will offer you a guaranteed income. In addition, you can usually negotiate a good benefits package.

If you are an entrepreneur and enjoy the challenge and risks involved in owning your own business, you may want to try solo private practice. If you need to, you can almost always affiliate with at least one IPA or PPO. The rewards of solo practice are many: You are in complete control of your professional life; you can, in the right setting, make lots of money; and you can establish traditional long-term patient relationships.

The Physician Employee of the Solo Practitioner

If their practices become too large to handle comfortably by themselves, solo practitioners may decide to hire other physicians as employees. The terms of these arrangements vary. In some the new physician is on a straight salary, in others the new physician receives a salary plus a bonus of some sort, and in still others the new physician receives a salary plus the option of eventually becoming a partner.

Arrangements for becoming a partner vary. After a predetermined time, you may be able to buy in for a set amount of money (usually paid over a number of years), or you may buy in through "sweat equity." Sweat equity is the equity you build up through your work. When you work for a salary, you usually generate more income than you receive. And some employers will count all or part of that extra income for a certain number of years as your buy in. The important thing in all these arrangements is that you understand *exactly* the terms of your employment and that you get a contract. (See Chapter IX.)

Being the employee of an established physician has many advantages in addition to those of being a solo practitioner. You have no start-up costs as well as none of the headaches of hiring staff and finding a facility. You can tap into an established patient base and referral network. You have on the spot a colleague and mentor with whom to talk over your cases. And you have the possibility of having your own practice or a partnership within a few years.

The disadvantages are more subtle. You may work very hard for a year or two and have little to show for your hard work but the salary you received. Also, unless you mesh well both personally and professionally with your employer, you may find that the tensions generated through different personal and professional styles outweigh any advantages. Often problems arise because young physicians probably know more about the latest developments in their fields and want to continue using all the new methods of treatment they were using during their residencies. Older physicians may resist the change and insist on their greater experience. But if both sides are willing to listen to and learn from each other, this type of arrangement can be profitable to both.

Shared Expenses

This practice type is exactly what it says. To help minimize costs, many times a physician will share a building, office staff, and equipment with one or more other physicians. They may even share some form of practice management and patient care. This practice type differs from a partnership or group because each physician's practice is technically a separate one, and each physician is still responsible for his or her own practice.

Partnership

A partnership exists when two or more physicians form a profit-making business in which they share both profits and liability equally or on some other predetermined basis. Like solo practitioners, they may or may not hire other physicians as salaried employees. And they may or may not give those physicians the option of becoming partners.

The advantages of being in a partnership are much the same as those of being in solo practice. You lose some control, but you have the advantage of shared expenses. Two physicians do not need twice as large a facility or support staff; one marketing campaign can include any number of physicians. Shared liability often means lower malpractice premiums and limited financial liability. And you have the benefit of collegiality—at least one other physician to consult with.

The disadvantages are much the same as those of being an employee of a solo practitioner. Many physicians compare partnerships to marriage, except that you spend more time with your partner or partners than you do with your spouse. Unless the personality mix is a good one, your professional life can become filled with tensions and problems that can create stress and detract from your practice of medicine.

Also, since a partnership is a business arrangement and most physicians are not businesspeople, problems can arise when the lines of command, responsibility, and income sharing have not been clearly drawn. So, for example, the physician who for whatever reason has taken over most of the administrative work may not receive any more income than the physician who just sees patients. The administrator-physician will probably begin to resent this increase in responsibility with no additional compensation.

Make sure you get professional help—at least an attorney and probably a practice management consultant—in drawing up a partnership agreement. And you must hire a business manager. But even hiring a business manager and an accountant does not relieve you of the responsibility of being aware of what is happening in your *business*. Business managers, accountants, and, indeed, even partners have been known to be dishonest. If the idea of having to keep tabs on a business appalls you, you would do well to consider being an employee.

Group

A group functions like a partnership except that to be called a group, you must have at least three physicians. Like the partnership, the group, a for-profit business, is organized formally and is a legal arrangement, with members sharing income, expenses, facilities, equipment, records, and personnel. Groups can be either single-specialty or multispecialty ones.

Although all the advantages and disadvantages of partnerships apply to groups, the problems are often compounded because of increased numbers of physicians and, in large multispecialty groups especially, of ancillary services provided. Income sharing, types of responsibility, the amount of power of each physician, how productivity is determined—

all must be clearly defined. Successful groups can have no gray areas. The psychiatrist in a multispecialty group, for example, must understand exactly how and why the ophthalmologist will probably be receiving a larger share of the group's income: Procedures earn more money.

The Physician Employee of a Partnership or of a Group

Partnerships and groups, especially large ones, often hire young doctors as employees, usually under the same terms the solo practitioner does. Also, the same advantages and disadvantages of the employees of solo practitioners apply to the employees of partnerships or groups. But in large groups, a young physician may feel more like an employee. You will have little or no say in the day-to-day running of the practice, you will have to learn to work in what is essentially a corporate setting, and you will probably have to wait longer to participate in profit sharing or to become a partner.

Open-Panel Model HMO (IPA or Network) or PPO

Open-panel model HMOs and PPOs are not practice types. They are contractual arrangements, which solo practitioners, partnerships, or groups may enter for the delivery of health care. They enter largely for two reasons: to protect or develop their patient base and to secure guaranteed payment for their services. Physicians participating in them practice in their own offices and have their own private practices. Also, they may belong to more than one plan. Thus, their income may derive from regular fee-for-service payment from private patients, from government reimbursement under Medicare and Medicaid, and from capitation payment from various IPAs or PPOs.

Open-Panel Model HMOs

The two forms of open-panel model HMOs are the network and the IPA. A network consists of two or more groups of physicians which agree to provide services to HMO members for a negotiated rate, usually fee-for-service but sometimes capitated. An IPA is a network of individual physicians, partnerships, and/or groups contracted to an administrative organization which agrees to provide services to its members at a prepaid, capitated rate. The providers, however, are paid at a negotiated fee-for-service rate. (See Figure 3 for an example of a typical IPA structure.)

The main advantages to the providers are a guaranteed cash flow and the preservation of their patient base. As the marketing director of a large IPA on the East Coast said, "When [a large corporation] signed on with us, we saw a huge influx of physicians. They weren't joining because they thought we were a great idea. They were joining because they were afraid of losing their patients. We're the lesser of two evils: They don't join, their patients go to docs who do, and they lose everything; they do join, their patients stay, and they get a pretty good percentage of their ordinary fee-for-service rate. They even pick up patients because of the increased referral base. And they know we're good pay."

Although they allow physicians to develop traditional long-term patient relationships and to practice independently, IPAs have certain disadvantages. Some financial risk is involved because a certain

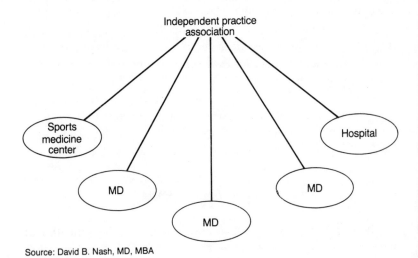

Source: David B. Nash, MD, MBA

Figure 3

percentage of physicians' fees are put into a "withhold pool" for covered tests and procedures. If, at the end of a set time, the pool is not large enough to pay for covered services, the physicians' fees are reduced accordingly. Money left in the pool at the end of that time, however, is divided equally among the providers.

The paperwork is voluminous. Physicians cannot refer their IPA patients to specialists outside the IPA. If they do, the patient must pay the fees. IPAs have no built-in consultation network or peer review. With everyone working independently, the collegiality of a true group does not exist, and control over quality of care is difficult to maintain.

Two other problems—one for the patient and one for the physician— are often shoved under the carpet. The first is that IPA patients sometimes may not receive the same quality of care as traditional patients. As Nash says, "The physician is running behind schedule. In examining room A is Mrs. Jones, the traditional patient. In examining room B is Mr. Smith, the IPA patient. Which one is going to get more time and attention? It's only human. And a lot of it is unconscious."

The other problem is what Nash calls the "angry, entitled patient." And this problem exists in all prepaid plans. Angry, entitled patients are almost always people who have been unemployed and through changed circumstances suddenly find themselves with jobs and benefits, including medical benefits. To this point, the patients' sole contact with the medical profession has been through emergency rooms or clinics. The patients do not know how to make appointments. But they know that they are entitled to health care—even in the middle of the night. So the patients call their primary-care physician at three a.m. because Sissy or Sonny is crying and is probably sick. And they want health care—now. If the patients do not get what they are "entitled" to, they become angry. In effect, these patients treat physicians like employees—something that many tired and harried young physicians find difficult to cope with.

PPOs

What is poetry? If you can answer that question in a few terse, pithy sentences, you can probably answer this one: What is a PPO? In their book, *PPOs Preferred Provider Organizations: An Executive's*

Guide, Samuel Tibbitts and Allen Manzano say, "Defining a PPO is like slicing batter, for the PPO cake has yet to be baked," and then develop a working definition:

> A [PPO] is a health financing and delivery arrangement in which a group of health care providers offers its services on a predetermined financial basis to health care purchasers under terms which encourage selection of the providers as the source of services to sponsored individuals.

They also quote the AHA's definition, which they think is too narrow:

> [A PPO is] a payment arrangement where insurers contract with hospitals or physicians on a fee-for-service basis to provide health care services. Subscribers can select any provider for care but they are given economic or other incentives to use these designated hospitals or physicians.

Nash defines PPOs as "any care delivery system that has a contractual arrangement with another system." In an article in the April 1987 issue of Piedmont Airlines' magazine, J. R. Gerson and Kenneth Friedenreich define PPOs as "a less formal [than HMOs] association of health care providers who agree to a fee schedule and receive reimbursement on a basis of fee for service."

Obviously, PPO is a term that is used generally to cover a variety of contractual arrangements with built-in cost and utilization procedures. (See Figure 4 for an example of a typical PPO structure.) These arrangements offer a discount to purchasers and a guaranteed share of the health-care market to providers. Because they are reimbursed less if they go to providers outside the PPO, subscribers have a vested interest in using only PPO providers. Among the providers are always physicians and hospitals.

For physicians, the advantages of affiliating with a PPO are maintenance of their patient base, of the traditional doctor-patient relationships, of their fee schedules, of a referral network, and of professional autonomy. Also, they can refer their patients to specialists and can order tests and procedures without worrying about costs coming out of their share of the pool. Because of peer review, PPOs offer more quality control than IPAs, so physicians sometimes feel more comfortable with the level

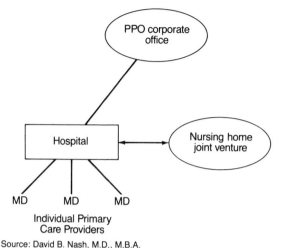

Source: David B. Nash, M.D., M.B.A.

Figure 4

of care their patients will receive from other providers in the plan. The primary disadvantage is—again—paperwork and having to work within set reimbursement schedules for tests and procedures.

Closed-Panel HMOs

Closed-panel HMOs, both group and staff models, are practice types. In the group model a group of physicians contracts with an HMO to provide medical services at a predetermined capitated rate. In the staff model, the HMO employs the physicians directly. In both models, patients must go to physicians in the HMO or must pay out of pocket if they do not.

The advantages of being in a closed-panel HMO are many. You have a built-in consulting network and a collegial atmosphere because everyone works as partners. Although bosses exist, they are not evident. The in-house peer review is less threatening than a more impersonal one. In a large HMO, you have access to labs and state-of-the-art equipment.

Perhaps the greatest advantages for the young physician are personal. You have no start-up costs, no practice management costs, no malpractice. You have a guaranteed salary (and sometimes a bonus or incentive plan) and good benefits package. In an article in the January 1987 issue of *Options*, Dan Gordon says, "These plans generally offer... comprehensive medical, dental, life, and long-term disability insurance; participation in a pension plan; an annual CME stipend of approximately $1,000, with five to ten days of travel time; paid professional organization dues; and vacations up to four weeks. Some also provide car allowances, paid moving expenses, profit-sharing plans, and stock options."

Also, you have set working hours and are seldom on call. In the same article, Gordon quotes Laura Rollins, program director of the AMA's practice management department, as saying that some people think "HMO should stand for 'home more often.'" One disadvantage is that because your regular hours might not include rounds, you might work a long day.

Among other disadvantages is the paperwork. Nash says, "Every consult, every lab test is a purchase order. They make it difficult to complete the forms, so physicians might limit tests." His statement points to another problem. Some people believe that the emphasis on cost containment affects the quality of care. All major national studies, however, show that this assumption is not true.

Patient care is often impersonal, with little opportunity to establish long-term patient relationships. Some HMOs limit the time physicians may spend with patients. Many HMO physicians feel as if they are part of a physician production line, seeing up to thirty or forty patients every day.

Also, the corporate structure of HMOs throws many new physicians off stride. Because they have never learned the unwritten corporate rules, they must spend time learning them on the job. Most physicians are good at taking tests and answering questions, not at playing corporate power games. In staff model HMOs particularly, physicians often begin to feel like hired hourly employees, with strict role definition and loss of autonomy.

Because of the drawbacks of practice in closed-panel HMO models, the turnover rate among entry-level physicians is relatively high. The average term of employment is two years. Still, many people coming out of residency see those two or three years as a chance to catch their breath before taking on the responsibilities of private practice, to pay off some of or all their medical school debts, and to get a better idea of how and where they want to practice medicine. If you do decide to become an HMO employee, be sure to have an attorney look over your contract and advise you about what you are agreeing to.

Institutional

Many physicians choose to become employees of institutions whose primary purpose is providing health care or which provide health care as a benefit to members or employees. Among the former are hospitals, especially government hospitals such as the Veterans' Administration (VA) system, ACCs or UCCs, nursing homes, and extended care facilities. Among the latter are schools, prisons, retirement centers, and corporations.

Most of these operate much like the closed-panel, staff model HMO. The physicians are employees with a good salary and benefits, set vacation time, regular call. They have no start up costs or malpractice costs and do not have to bother with what Nash calls the "business of practice." Often, in government institutions especially, the physician is able to treat patients without regard to cost of treatment. And in all these settings the physician is able to treat patients without regard to payment. Particularly in schools and corporations, the physician can often establish relatively long-term patient relationships and can become involved in preventive medicine and in developing health and safety programs.

One of the disadvantages of this type of practice is the relatively lower income level compared with that of physicians in private practice. In some of these settings, the physician is relatively isolated from colleagues so loses the collegiality of group practice. Also the physician has little or no control over the clinical environment. Because of the bureaucratic red tape that often goes along with this type of practice setting, making changes is often difficult or impossible. The frustration level can be quite high. If you try to upset the status quo, you might be seen as a troublemaker. Sometimes the administration of these institutions is in an adversarial position to the physicians. Also, while their perception is almost always incorrect, many people in the medical profession see these

physician-employees as less competent than their entrepreneur colleagues. As a result, moving from this type of practice may be difficult.

The Military

The military is the country's largest HMO. (The VA is second.) If
you are considering the military as a career option, you are probably
already involved with the military in some way. You may have been
in R.O.T.C. as an undergraduate. You may be a graduate of the Uni-
form Services Health Science University. You may be involved in
one of the military residency programs. In any case, you most likely
know by now exactly what your commitment is to the military.

The advantages and disadvantages of military practice are exactly
the same as those in institutional practice. In the military, though,
you would probably have better benefits and more collegiality. Also
you would have a much freer hand in ordering tests and procedures
for your patients and in referring them to specialists.

Academia

Most of you, after all these years in academia, understand how
academic medicine works, and you already know most of the advantages and disadvantages. Two of the disadvantages that you may
not have considered, however, are that getting to the top in academic
medicine is often very difficult and that to move up you often have
to move. On average, physicians in academic medicine move more
often than other physicians.

If you decide to explore an academic position, carefully determine
exactly what your responsibilities would be. How much time must
you allocate to teaching? To research? To administrative work? Are
you able to have your own private practice, or are you expected to
be just a salaried employee? Is the position you are considering a
tenure-track one? What kind of support will you get for research?
The answers to these questions vary from institution to institution.

Research

You may by now have decided that you do not really want to practice medicine, that you want to do research. Although you can do research in academic medicine, you also have to have some sort of direct patient care. But in corporations and in the government, you can often just do research.

Again, you will be an employee, with all that that implies. And, in the government especially, you will have to cope with red tape and forms. Although government research, like academic research, is pure research, you should understand that corporate research is powered by the profit motive. You will be expected to make money for your employer. If you do decide to go into research in any setting, make sure you have clarified what happens to your discoveries. Do they belong to you or to your employer?

Other Opportunities

As medicine becomes more and more big business, many opportunities exist in administrative and managerial work, both in the government and with large corporate health-care providers. Also as medicine becomes more technologically complicated, pharmaceutical and other medical supply companies are adding physicians to their staffs, especially in sales and sales support. If you are attracted by the idea of becoming a physician-executive, you might want to explore some of these opportunities.

Just as you did in assessing your needs, you will have to consider all your options for practice opportunities and then decide which ones best fit your needs right now and how they fit with your long-term goals. Once you have decided which practice types or settings appeal most to you, find out as much as you can about them—before you begin your job search. The more information you have ahead of time, the more successful the search will be.

Chapter VI

Assessing Your Value

Now that you have determined the job you want, you should determine your chances of getting it. Assessing your value in the marketplace is difficult. You have to decide the relative worth of many things in your background, training, and credentials: AMG versus FMG, M.D. versus D.O., Board Certified versus Board Eligible, the reputation of your training program, your experience and specific hard skills, your soft skills. There are so many things to consider that you may want to give up before you even begin. But this part of your job search is important. If you set unreasonably high expectations for the type of job and the amount of the compensation you can get, you will doom yourself to a dissatisfying job search.

If you are not sure what constitutes reasonable expectations, ask people. Sit down with your chairperson or your attendings and ask for help in assessing your value in the market. They can often provide information about practice opportunities and compensation in your specialty. And they can help you assess your strengths and weaknesses.

Another good way to approach the problem is to make up a chart of your qualifications and the requirements of the job and to fill it in with pluses and minuses. Adding up your pluses and minuses will let you see how you measure up and will give you some idea of whether you are being realistic. The most important thing is that you try to be realistic about yourself. Do not overvalue—or undervalue—yourself.

YOUR CREDENTIALS

Although everyone knows that CVs tell relatively little about a person, everyone also knows that people use CVs as a tool to whittle down the number of candidates for a job. As one chairman said, "When I see a CV with Stanford, Chicago, Pennsylvania, Mayo, I know the candidate has something. I want to bring him or her in so I can get a closer look." Unless you get a personal referral for the job you want, your credentials are your foot in the door.

AMG versus FMG

One of the first things you will be judged on is whether you are an American medical graduate. In today's competitive marketplace, AMGs have an edge on FMGs. If, however, you are an FMG who has gone through a good residency program and if you have built a good network, the people hiring may overlook your FMG status. Conversely, if you are a one hundred percent AMG but have the personality of a fish, your AMG status will not offset your bad references.

In the eyes of people hiring, the greatest drawback for FMGs is not their knowledge or technical skills but often their communication skills. Even if your reading and writing skills are good, your verbal skills are what will determine your value in the marketplace. You must be able to understand the innuendos of *American* English. Can you understand jokes? Can you understand your patients who use slang or colloquialisms when they are describing their problems? Do you pick up the subtle differences in intonation?

If your answer to any one of these questions is no, you should—as soon as possible—study conversational American English. And one British FMG recommends that you try to take some courses in American culture. Understanding the culture will help you understand not only the unconscious assumptions of your colleagues and patients but also the subtleties of the language.

Do not take one more course in formal standard English—you have already done that. You need to learn how to speak American English, even if your native language is British or Australian English. Everyone has heard the stories of misunderstandings between "English"-speaking people—the American who thinks he is being offered something quite different from a wake up call when his British landlady asks if he would like a "knockup" in the morning or the Australian who thinks the American is being too open when he says, "Hi, I'm Randy."

If you cannot find a class in American English conversation, try to find someone who will work with you. Actually, one-on-one conversation is much more efficient and effective than group conversation when learning to speak another language. In groups everyone is at a different level, so you cannot work as intensively as you should to prepare yourself for the job market.

You might try what one Japanese physician did—go to a speech pathologist at your hospital. He asked for help from the head of the speech pathology department where he was training, and the chairperson suggested that he get in touch with one of the pathologists who was interested in learning as many foreign languages as she could. The pathologist and the physician traded skills. She taught him colloquial English, telling him jokes and using slang, and he taught her rudimentary Japanese, enough so that the next summer she could travel comfortably in Japan. In only three months of half-hour sessions five or six times a week, his verbal skills had improved so dramatically that his chairperson called him in to ask how he had learned to speak American English so quickly and so well. An added benefit—while he was learning to speak "American," the physician had made a good friend too. And the whole thing cost him nothing but his time.

Even if you do learn to speak colloquially and if you come from a good residency program, you should be prepared for a difficult job search. Everyone knows that many FMGs are among the finest physicians in the country—in teaching, in research, and in patient care. Because of the competitive marketplace, however, some FMGs must struggle for good jobs.

When asked if he would hire an FMG, one chairperson at a large regional medical center began to explain that of course he would if the person had good credentials, could speak well, was personable. But when pressed, when asked what would happen if he had two fairly equal candidates but one was an AMG and the other an FMG, he looked over his glasses and said, "Would you like to know the reality? We have one FMG, and he's here because he not only has excellent credentials but he also has a relative on the staff. The problem is not with the quality of the FMGs but with people's—and I mean lots of the people in medicine's—perception of them. Physicians tend to think, 'Oh, with all those FMGs, they must not have a good program. They must not be able to attract good doctors.' It's not pleasant, but there it is."

Another drawback for FMGs is the licensing requirements of different states. Almost all have special requirements for foreign medical graduates. So if you decide you want to practice in a specific area, be sure to check them out ahead of time. One American FMG had actually accepted a job and gone to the town, only to discover that he had to wait a year before he could even apply for a license.

M.D. versus D.O.

If your degree is in osteopathic medicine, your chances in the job market may not be as good as they would be if your degree were in allopathic medicine. If you did your residency in an allopathic program, your chances may be better. But even then you should realize that many people—in medicine—have antiquated ideas about osteopathic training. In fact, they may confuse you with a chiropractor.

In considering a job, you should try to determine how comfortable the community and the physicians on the staff are with the idea of osteopathy. If you are the first osteopath on the medical staff and if the staff is an old-boy network of M.D.s, you will have to work hard to gain credibility as a good doctor and to build your patient base. Not that you will not be able to do these things. You just need to be aware that you have to be better than the best, that is if you get the job at all. Many people have absolutely closed their minds to osteopathy. One search committee refused even to consider a D.O., in spite of his having better credentials and training than the M.D. candidates. Their reason: "We've never had one on our staff."

Another reason that people may be reluctant to hire you is that they may be suspicious of your loyalties. Say, for example, that you are being considered by an allopathic hospital in a community that has an osteopathic hospital. The people hiring may be afraid that after they help you establish your practice, your emotional ties to osteopathy will eventually pull you to the osteopathic hospital. Realistic? No. Reality? Yes.

You should also check the licensing rules of the states you would like to practice in to see if they have special requirements for D.O.s.

Even having your board certification may not be enough if you are certified in osteopathic medicine even though some of you have trained longer and even though your exams are certainly as rigorous. One retiring M.D. said, "You know, they [osteopaths] are trying all kinds of things to circumvent the system. The next thing you know we'll be having podiatrists apply for certification." That too is the reality.

One happy note is that many people are beginning to realize the value of your manipulative training, especially in specialties such as physiatry and orthopedics. As a result, in some instances you might have an edge on your M.D. competitors. Also, many people hiring are paying more attention to the traditional osteopathic concern with the whole patient. One pediatrician with a degree in osteopathy got his job because the group hiring him—all M.D.s—was impressed with his holistic approach to patient care.

Board Certified versus Board Eligible

Obviously, you will be in a much better bargaining position if you are on the board certification track. Medicine is so competitive now that many hospitals will not even consider someone who is not either board certified or within a year or two of certification. Many contracts now stipulate that you must be board certified within a specific number of years. As one hospital CEO put it, rather callously, "One good thing for us about the oversupply [of physicians] in this area is that we're able to work on upgrading our medical staff. We can be a lot more demanding about things like certification."

So if you are not board certified or on your way to being so, you may have to think about going to an area that is underserved. Or if you want to stay in a metropolitan area, you may have to consider a city public hospital.

Your Medical School and Training Program

People will be judging you, initially anyway, on the prestige of your medical school and especially on the prestige of your training program. In fact, if you went to a well known medical school but ended up in a small program in a remote area, people may think something is wrong. A chairperson of cardiology said, "When I get the CV, and it says Ohio State Medical School and Podunk training program, now that sets off warning bells in my mind. I think to myself that this person must not have been a very good medical student because coming out of Ohio State if the person was good, he'd be able to go to a better place than Podunk."

The reverse is also true. If you went to a mediocre medical school but ended up in a nationally known program, people will think you must be a superstar. The same chairperson said, "Now when I see Podunk medical school and Baylor training program, I'm impressed right away. For a person to get from Podunk to Baylor, he'd have to be very good indeed. I'd probably call around, and if everything else checked out, I'd want to bring him in for an interview."

If neither your medical school nor your training program is particularly well known, you may have a more difficult time getting a job than people who went to prestigious schools and training programs. A kind of snobbery develops in people who did go through the best programs. They often feel that people out of other programs do not quite measure up. You probably do, but unless you have a strong network, you may not have the chance to prove you do, especially if you are in a competitive specialty and want to go to a medical mecca.

However, some people are beginning to reassess the old assumptions. The head of surgery at a fine, small community hospital on the East Coast said, "It used to be that you always went after the people from Harvard or Columbia or places like that. The idea was that having them on your staff gave you greater prestige. But we haven't liked some of the things we've seen in a few of the people from those high powered programs. The programs are so competitive they're more like intellectual warfare than education. That cutthroat competitiveness carries over.

"We had a guy here one summer who gave other people in the program misinformation—you know, telling them they didn't have to come in for certain things, like lectures, and then he'd be the only one here, just so he'd look better. He applied for a job with us. But we weren't interested. Of course we wouldn't consider anyone who wasn't a skilled surgeon. But these days we're trying to look past the credentials for the human qualities."

Being the chief resident in your program, no matter what its reputation, is a plus for you. People will automatically see you as a leader and as a good organizer and administrator. They will assume that you have the best combination of hard and soft skills of all the people in your year. If you were in a program in which the chief residency rotated among all of you, you do not have to say so on your CV—just Chief Resident and the year—especially if you trained in a less well known program. You are not lying. That information can come out later, in the interview. Remember you need a foot in the door.

Fellowship Training

Having done a fellowship is also a plus. People see you as committed to continued growth and development in your field. A chairperson in a major teaching hospital said, "When I see a fellowship there on the CV, that tells me the person wants to know as much as he can. He wants to be the best he can. That's the kind of thing we're looking for. Medicine today is changing and growing so much and is so specialized that there's not room in a program like ours for the person who is content just to complete the basic training requirements and then go out and practice—you know, the type who just does minimum CME year in and year out.

Doing fellowship training in a good, well known program is one way to offset a less well known residency training program. And it certainly expands your network. Among other benefits of fellowship training is its effect on your first-year compensation. Estimates suggest that a fellowship can add twenty to twenty-five percent to the basic package.

Special Skills and Experience

If during your training you have had the opportunity to learn and to practice highly specialized procedures, you will be in a much better position than someone in your field who has not. For one thing, procedures make money for you and for your employers or partners. For another, in their effort to compete for their share of the market, hospitals are constantly trying to expand their services and, as a result, need physicians who can perform the latest procedures. So if you have done lots of MRI work, for example, you will be a valuable asset to a hospital that is trying to get approval to add an MRI to its radiology department.

In some instances, however, broader-based training is an asset. Many groups and good, small community hospitals need utility players, people who have had experience performing a wider variety of routine procedures. So if you have had the opportunity to be the primary surgeon in a number of different types of operations, for example, you will be a valuable asset to a hospital that is looking for a replacement for a retiring general surgeon.

YOUR REFERENCES

One important thing you need to consider in assessing your value in the job market is the quality of your references. Quality here does not necessarily mean the reputation of the people writing letters for you. Of course, if you have assisted a leader in your field who thinks you are the hottest thing to hit medicine since antibiotics, you are going to be an excellent candidate. But most people agree that having good letters from people who know you and who have worked closely with you is better than having neutral letters from nationally known people who may have seen you only in passing.

Quality here means the quality of the reference itself. What will people say about you? Although one bad reference will not put you out of the running for a job, it will make people try to get a broader and deeper picture of you. In an effort to put the bad, or even so-so, reference into context, they will call people they know who have worked with you— peers, attendings, ancillary staff—even though you may not have listed them as references. They will also call the references you have listed and ask much more probing questions about you and your work.

You can see that knowing what your references *really* think of you is important. Some people might be able to write a perfectly good letter about you. But if they have reservations or concerns about either your work or your personality, those things will come out in the telephone calls.

Also, if you give as references people who do not think very highly of you or your work, you will mark yourself as someone who does not have a clear picture of who he or she is. For example, a search consultant called a reference who began by saying, "I can't imagine why he gave my name." In the course of the call, the consultant asked the reference's opinion of the physician's mental stability. The reply? "Oh, marginal." Obviously, the consultant immediately dismissed the physician as a candidate—not because of his "marginal" mental stability (that could have been the misconception of someone who did not much like him) but because of his lack of self-awareness.

Also, put what your references will say about you into the context of the type of job you want. References are often asked to rank you on a scale of one to ten. You do not have to be a ten across the board to get a good job. If you are coming out of a program such as the Mayo Clinic's and your chairperson ranks you as a six in research, that six will not matter if you want to go into a group or community-based hospital and practice medicine. But if you want to stay in academic medicine, that six may present problems. It may not really be high enough to get you a good academic job.

If you receive low rankings across the board in clinical competency, however, you will not be in a very strong position in the job market. You should seriously reassess your chances for getting the kind of job you want. You may have to take a job in a geographic area or in a professional environment you may not want. Remember that people expect clinical competency.

The same is as true personally as professionally. No matter how strong your clinical skills, if your people skills are weak, you will have a difficult time finding a job. But, again, you do not need tens across the board. In doing a reference check on a physician, for example, a search consultant found that all her references ranked her at ten for her diagnostic skills. But they gave her only a five for efficiency. She was so methodical in her diagnosing that she took a long time with each patient. So while she was not suited to a job where she would be the only person in her specialty or where she would be working as part of a team, she was an excellent candidate for a job where she would be one of a group of people in her specialty, where she could take her time on the more difficult cases and make the diagnoses that might elude some of her colleagues.

You have to put all these things into context. Getting a five or six because you are shy and introverted will not be a minus if you are applying for a job where you can work in the background or where you will not be expected to help your group's public relations. But getting a five or six because you are arrogant and rude will be a minus no matter what kind of job you apply for.

Some of you might echo the resident who asked, "How does anyone know if he's arrogant? Isn't lack of awareness part of the pattern?" If you are a good physician, you should be sensitive and empathetic. If you are sensitive and empathetic, you understand your effect on people. If you have no clue about your effect on the people around you—to paraphrase Hippocrates—physician, know thyself. And if, in coming to know yourself, you discover that the people you work with have a more negative view of you than you thought, heal thyself—before the job search.

PERSONAL CONSIDERATIONS

You need to look at any personal pluses or minuses that will affect your chances of finding the job you want. Pluses such as having a degree in another field or having business experience can increase your value—especially in modern medicine where the physician is often expected to be an entrepreneur or to be able to thread the legal labyrinths of tax laws and government regulations. Minuses such as having a history of substance abuse or having a poor personal appearance can decrease your value. Your race or your sex can also affect your value when you apply for certain kinds of jobs.

Experience Outside Medicine

Although you might think that being older than most of your peers when you enter the medical job market will be a minus, having experience in other fields will actually give you an edge on your younger colleagues and will often balance negative factors in your background. For one thing, your work in another field will enhance your work in medicine. For another, potential employers will see you as settled, mature, and committed to your work. People who turn to medicine after having worked in other fields know what they want to do.

A hospital CEO said, "When I see teaching or counseling or sales on CVs, I look at those people differently. They're going to bring to the job special skills—whether they're people or entrepreneurial skills or both—that people who have spent their lives just in medicine won't have. I feel just a little more confident about those people. I know that I won't have to hold their hands."

Medicine today is big business. But most physicians, immersed in their own work, are not businesspeople. As one physician said, "We're the easiest mark around for investment sharks or dishonest bookkeepers or accountants. For all we know about medicine, we don't have a clue about business." Hospitals and groups are looking for physicians with business experience or M.B.A.s or law degrees.

One older family medicine physician, for example, thought he would have a difficult time finding a job. He had been a conscientious objector during the Vietnam War. But instead of leaving the country or going to jail, he asked the draft board to give him another job that would take the place of military service and ended up doing inner-city social work in New York for four years. After that, he worked successfully in insurance and real estate sales.

In the midst of making piles of money, he reassessed his life and decided he wanted to work with people again, as a doctor. Because of his age and background, he had to go to a foreign medical school and, as a result, was unable to go into a first-rate training program. Everything seemed to be against him.

But instead of scrambling for a job, he found himself with a number of job offers. The group he finally went to work for chose him over many other "better qualified" candidates. Because the group's focus was on holistic medicine and on treating the whole family, the other physicians thought that his experience in social work would make him more attuned to family needs. And they needed his entrepreneurial skills.

Substance Abuse

If you have a history of substance abuse, even though you may be rehabilitated, you will have a more difficult time finding a job than a physician who does not. Whether or not to mention the problem before the interview is the subject of much debate. Some people believe that you should be open about the problem from the beginning, but most people seem to think that while you should not mention it in letters of application or on the CV, you should bring it up in the interview.

A chairperson of medicine said, "To be perfectly honest, if I see anything about chemical dependency, or if I hear about it before I meet the person, I'd never consider the candidate. There are too many good people out there to take that kind of chance. But if I like everything about the person and he or she brings up the problem in the interview—you know the sort of thing, 'Well, now that we've been talking for a while, there's one thing I do need to tell you. I fudged a bit. . . .'—then the monkey's on my back, so to speak. As a physician, I'm supposed to be understanding."

If you do have a problem with substance abuse right now, do not think you will be able to hide it. Even though you might be able to find a job now, the problem will surface as it begins to get worse (it always does) and as you begin to work closely with your colleagues. Then you will probably lose your job for lying in the first place, and you will destroy your network.

Do something about the problem right away. As a physician, you know it is not going to go away by itself. Find a rehabilitation program that works primarily with physicians and that will act as your advocate in the job market. People working in a program of this sort are more aware of the special needs of physicians. They understand the pressure cooker that physicians live in, which many times drives physicians to alcohol or drugs as an escape. And the advocacy of the physicians in the program will lend credibility to your rehabilitation.

Physical Appearance

For a physician, obesity may be a handicap. Obesity suggests many things to potential employers—none of them good. It suggests that you lack discipline—and if you are undisciplined, you probably will not be an effective doctor. It suggests that you do not care about yourself—and if you do not care about yourself, you probably will not care much about anything else. It suggests that you are not health-oriented—and if you disregard the latest medical information about the effects of obesity, you probably will not pay much attention to the latest medical information about anything.

Although none of these perceptions may be true of you, you should be realistic about the fact that many people will see you this way. Also, you must face the fact that your obesity may interfere in your patient relationships. Many people, for example, do not like to be touched by obese people. And your patients may not take you seriously as a physician. How will you be able to tell them to quit smoking, get into an exercise program, or lose weight when you so obviously do not follow your own advice? If you are obese, try to begin working on your problem before you start your job search.

One resident who weighed over two hundred pounds found that everyone—attendings, peers, patients—ignored her. They seemed literally not to see her. On rounds her attendings never asked her questions. The other residents never talked to her about the patients or difficult cases. Her patients always checked what she said with nurses or other physicians. So she decided to change her image. She lost more than a hundred pounds, had her hair cut and styled, and bought a new wardrobe. She says, "It was as if a new doctor suddenly appeared in their midst. I had authority where before I had none." Today, she is a department head in a well known teaching program.

Looking unkempt or, worse, dirty is another handicap for physicians. In your work, you must be meticulous, careful, neat, and clean. You must be the same in your appearance. You may have impeccable work habits, but if you are sloppy looking, no one will believe you do. If you do not care about your appearance, people will assume you do not care about your work.

In a close call between herself and another physician, one physician did not get a job because she had dandruff. The head of the search committee said, "When she was nervous, which was most of the day, she kept rubbing the side of her head. And a great cloud of dandruff would drift down to her shoulder. All I could think about was how I'd feel if I were her patient. I couldn't stand it. By the end of the day, I

didn't even want to go to dinner with her. It's not just the physical re-
pulsiveness either. Why didn't she *do* something about it?'' If your appearance is a mess, do something about it. Unlike problems such as
chemical dependency or obesity, this one can be solved fairly easily.

Sex, Race, and Ethnic Background

In a perfect world none of these things would matter. In our de-
cidedly imperfect world, they do. The situation is improving, but if
you are a woman, if you are black, if you are Jewish, if you are Hispanic—if you are anything other than an "American" male physician, you might find yourself in situations where your sex or race or
ethnic background will put you at a disadvantage in the job market.

Because they believe that women have too many loyalties outside medicine, some male physicians are reluctant to hire women.
Men are afraid that if women are married, they will follow their hus-
bands if they change jobs, or if women are not married, they will get
married and do the same thing. Men are afraid that women with children will be torn between the demands of motherhood and of the
profession. One physician said, "The influx of women into medicine,
especially married ones with children, is turning it into a nine-to-five
profession—and it's not. It can't be." Although they see evidence all
around them that women physicians are just as hard working and
dedicated as their male colleagues, the reality is that some male physicians ignore the evidence and cling to the notion that being a wife
and mother and being a physician are mutually exclusive.

Some men also believe that because of their "conflicts" between
family and job, women are more likely to have psychological problems than men are. And some men still believe that while women
are "okay for routine cognitive work," only men can be trusted with
highly complex procedures. So you need to realize that even though
you may be the hardest working, most stable, brightest, and skilled
physician in your program, some potential employers will be unable
to see you as you really are. They will be unable to move beyond
their picture of the female physician.

The same is true if you are black or Hispanic. No matter what your record and accomplishments, some physicians will never be able to believe that you are really competent. If you are Jewish, physicians in some areas of the country will believe that you would be too abrasive or aggressive to work well in their groups. People hire in their own image—and the image outside of major metropolitan areas is not usually minority or ethnic.

Obviously, many physicians have let go of the old stereotypes. And even if they have not yet been able to quite let go of them, they are trying, so they will give you a fair shot at the job. You just need to be aware that in certain situations "what" you are will be a minus.

In some instances, the people hiring may themselves not have a problem with your sex, race, or background. But they may feel that the community would have problems accepting a physician who is "different." Because they want to succeed and they want the physician they bring in to succeed, they might decide against you.

Sometimes, however, "what" you are will be a plus. One group in a community with a large Hispanic blue-collar population asked a search consultant specifically to find a Hispanic physician to replace its retiring pediatrician. Why? Because they wanted to tap into that market. Blue-collar patients are generally considered to be the easiest to deal with and the quickest to pay their doctor bills.

YOUR DOLLAR VALUE

Many of you hear stories of people who earn six-figure incomes in their first year of practice, and you immediately assume that you will do the same. Probably you will not. That six-figure income may be based on many factors that do not apply to you. The person earning that salary may have been the number one person in the number one training program. Or the person may have accepted a job in a place you would not even think of going to. Or the person may be in a field in which first-year guarantees are higher across the board than those in your specialty. For example, first-year OB/GYNs can expect to earn somewhere between $60,000 and $75,000 but first-year orthopedic surgeons can expect $85,000 to $125,000. Other specialties range somewhere in between.

Another reason your figures may be off is that the new Internal Revenue Service ruling on tax-exempt institutions is changing the compensation packages that hospitals are offering first-year physicians. Hospital administrators need to show that your coming into the community will benefit the hospital. So, in an effort not to hurt their tax-exempt status, hospitals are moving from offering first-year guarantees and free office space and staff support to offering more or less straight salaries. With a salary, they can demonstrate that you work so many hours per day per week for them.

Before you begin your job search, you should have a fairly clear picture of what kind of offer you will be willing to accept. Do research on starting salaries in your specialty in the geographic area you want. Your research can be as informal as calling people you know and asking. Or you can look through journals such as *Medical Economics, JAMA,* and the *AMA News.* About once a year, journals such as these publish articles about physician compensation by specialty and often by geographic area. Once you get some general idea of the range in your area, average the first-year consult salary with the first-year guarantee, or flat salary. The figure you come up with should be a good starting point for you when you are trying to determine a realistic salary.

Do not forget that compensation may include everything from malpractice insurance to mortgage assistance to equipment and supplies. Once you have an idea of the range of starting salaries in your specialty and in the geographic area you want, you should determine what other benefits you need: Will you need help with malpractice insurance? With relocating expenses? (For a more detailed discussion of compensation packages, see Chapter IX, "Getting the Offer and Negotiating the Contract.") Decide what trade-offs you can make.

Through this process of assessing your value, remember that the key word is *realistic.* But if after all the talking and looking at your pluses and minuses, you really believe that you can do a job that everyone says you will not be able to do, try for it. Obviously, you should have other options—jobs that everyone says you will be able to do. But you know yourself better than anyone else does, and you might turn up a winner. You have nothing to lose.

Most people discourage first-year physicians from starting out in solo practice. If you know, however, that you are an entrepreneur, that you love business, or if you have been successful in business, go into solo practice. When her mentors questioned her decision to go immediately into solo practice, one physician who had worked in sales for almost ten years said, "Just give me the chance. I couldn't stand the humdrum life of an employee. I want to be my own boss. And I know I'll love it." She's been in practice for four years and is now looking for a partner because her patient load is so heavy she cannot manage it alone. She is happy too.

Another physician, a black OB/GYN, was urged not even to think about an opportunity in a small southern community. But he wanted to go back to the South, to his roots. Because they thought he would not be able to build up a strong patient base, the people in the community sponsoring the practice had strong reservations about bringing him in. And they even tried to discourage him by offering him a lower first-year guarantee than they would have offered a white physician. Although he had an offer in Chicago, he persisted and now, five years later, is the most successful OB/GYN in the area. His patients are both black and white.

As one patient said, "I know it sounds trite, but he has an incredible bedside manner. He makes you feel as if he really cares about you. And he listens. I had gone to a dermatologist for a rash that had spread from my face to my stomach around my waist and was moving down my legs. When I suggested that the problem could be a combination of stress and sulfur preservatives in food and too many eggs, the dermatologist smiled and said something about pine pollen. When I told Dr. [Jones], he listened carefully to my theory and even said it made sense. He talked to me about my stress and sent me to another dermatologist. I love Dr. Jones. We all do. I have to admit I was hesitant at first, but not any more."

So when all the charts are against you and people are telling you "Forget it!" remember the black male OB/GYN in the South. What odds could be more overwhelming? Yet he succeeded. You should be realistic about your value, but sometimes you also should take a chance on yourself.

Chapter VII

Marketing Yourself

Now that you have laid the groundwork—built a good network, determined what you want and how you want to practice, set realistic goals for yourself—you are ready to begin searching for a job. As you look at the number of possibilities available to you, you may feel overwhelmed. For most of your life, your choices have been relatively limited. When you went to high school, to college, to medical school, to your training program, you had only so many places to choose from.

Also, you had little trouble seeking out these places. You could find lists of colleges and medical schools in counselors' offices and bookstores. You could find lists of available residency programs through your medical school or in the AMA "green book." Now suddenly you are faced with boundless and often nebulous choices. How do you even begin to go about finding a job?

You can use either one or a combination of two major ways to find a job: you can market yourself through entrepreneurship and networking, by responding to ads, or through direct mail; or you can have someone else, a "head hunter," market you.

When do you begin? Usually in the summer before your last year of residency. Most people ideally want to have their jobs by December or January of their last year in training. Remember that you need lots of lead time before you actually begin your new job. Credentialing and licensing take at least a few months. Your spouse may have to find a job. You need to find a place to live. You may have to set up your practice.

Job searching is a time-consuming business. Even if you have done all your preliminary assessments, you still have to locate jobs, pursue them, and go to interviews—usually two for each job. And on average you will probably be looking at about ten jobs. Try to arrange your rotations in your last year so you will have time for everything.

Often you will have to use vacation time, or you will have to trade coverage with other residents.

If you have not determined your priorities—lifestyle, professional environment, money, practice type—and your value in the market, you will spend huge amounts of mostly unproductive time in your job search. You will become what people call a "job shopper." If you do become a job shopper, you may end up going to twenty or more interviews.

Not knowing what you want or where you want to go, you will spend a great deal of time following up all kinds of leads you really have no interest in, vacillating between choices, trying to find everything that is out there. Because the race is on, anxiety sets in, and you become the equivalent of an ambulance chaser—chasing down everything instead of chasing down the things that are real possibilities for you. And the more you chase, the more confused you become.

So make the time to define the kind of job you want and where you want it *before you begin to look!* You will save yourself and everyone else involved enormous amounts of time.

One very important piece of advice as you begin your job search: When you do identify a possible lead, keep the information to yourself. Medicine today is competitive. You may think that your fellow residents would not hurt you, and probably they would not. But remember that they need jobs too. Share your job leads *only* after you have disqualified them for yourself. Think about yourself first. Doing so is not being selfish; it is being smart.

One physician in her excitement about a possible job discussed it with a fellow resident with whom she had been very close friends all through training. When she interviewed, she found that the hospital was interviewing her friend as well. She was shocked: "You know, I couldn't believe he did that to me. He is my friend. And he knows that I don't have that much leeway in applying for jobs because my husband is still in residency, so we need to stay in the Boston area."

She had not counted on the fact that he would have his own agenda. He, too, wanted to stay in the Boston area, and medicine is particularly competitive in Boston. When she confronted him, he replied, "Look, if you get hired, I'll be happy for you. If I get hired, I'll be happy for me, and I'd think you would be too." She tried to make him understand her anger and sense of betrayal, but he countered by saying that someone else had really told him about the job.

Interestingly enough, neither physician got the job. Instead, a good friendship and a mutually supportive working relationship were destroyed. The two physicians were never more than polite to each other after the experience.

Before you can keep a lead to yourself, however, you have to find one. Where do you begin?

BEING AN ENTREPRENEUR

One way to begin your search is to keep track of every lead you hear about. A good idea is to keep a small notebook—one the pages will not fall out of—in which you jot down information about possible opportunities. Every time you hear about a group that is growing and thinking of adding someone in your specialty, an HMO that is opening in the area you want to practice in, a hospital that is expanding its services, write it down, even if you have to write it down on a napkin in the cafeteria. Just be sure to transfer it to your notebook later.

Begin to intertwine yourself in the network that is already established in the medical field. One exists even if you are not aware of it—among physicians, hospital administrators, HMO administrators, physician executives. By the time you are entering your last year of residency, you may have found three or four jobs that sound particularly interesting to you. When you have time, follow up your leads.

Right now, you may be saying to yourself, "Time? Where do I find the time to do anything else but my job?" Just as with determining the kind of job you want, where you want it, and your chances of getting it, making time now will save you from the panic and scramble of job searching at the end of training.

Often, by following up your leads, you will find the "hidden job market." You may find a job that no one else knows about because it has not opened yet or has not been publicized yet. You can be-

come a serious candidate before any others arrive on the scene—
because you will be a known quantity to the decision makers.

In his next to last year of residency when he was home visiting his
family, one physician, for example, heard about a hospital in the area
that had a certificate of need (CON) in for a twenty-bed inpatient rehabilitation unit. He wrote his information in his notebook and, when
he returned to training, got the name of the chief executive officer (CEO)
from the American Hospital Association Guide and wrote to him. The
physician said that while he was home, he had heard about the new
unit and that he would like to come in to talk to the CEO the next time
he was home. He did not say he wanted a job, just that he wanted to
talk.

About two or three weeks later he followed up the letter with a
phone call. The CEO told him that the CON had, in fact, been approved but that establishing the unit would take some time. He also
invited the physician to come in to talk with people at the hospital
because physical medicine and rehabilitation was a new field for them
and they would welcome information from someone training in the
field.

From marketing and demographic surveys the hospital had found
that the closest rehabilitation unit was more than one hundred miles
away and that the hospital's secondary service area had a population of
more than two hundred fifty thousand people. Because the hospital was
already an excellent, state-of-the-art community hospital, the administrators wanted to develop a rehabilitation unit that would not only maintain but also enhance the reputation of the hospital.

They talked to the physician about how to set up the unit and
staff it and about what kind of census they could expect the first year.
Although he said the first year's patient mix would probably be com-
prised mostly of stroke patients, he discussed ways of broadening
the program to include most disabilities. A few months later they called
him back to talk further about the development of the program.

One year later the physician opened that rehabilitation unit. He
had discovered the hidden job market. He had absolutely no competition for that job. No ad ever appeared in a journal. No other candidate was ever interviewed. He did not go in to ask for a job; he just

went in to talk. But somewhere along the way he had let them know he could do the job for them.

He laughs now about the fact that, although he obviously needed letters of reference to get his license and to be credentialed, he has never developed a CV: "If I make a job change, I don't know what I'll do about a CV. I've never prepared one." When asked what he would have done if that job had not worked out, since he had not followed any other leads, he said, "Oh, I would have gotten another job. It's just that it was exciting to get this one on my own initiative. Half the fun was going in there and selling myself to them, letting them see that I could do the job they needed to have done." What he did was risky in a way, but it was also entrepreneurial. And you need a little entrepreneurial spirit if you are going to find a job that is right for you.

For busy residents, however, entrepreneurship does have a couple of big drawbacks: It is time-consuming, and you hit many dead ends. You may call only to find that the job will not be available for another year. Or the people hiring may have already found someone for the job. Or they may be interviewing their "final" candidate: "We're already interviewing someone from XYZ program. If it doesn't work out, we'll get back to you. Please send us your CV." Occasionally, they get back to you. But in the meantime, you are left waiting for someone to respond to you. And waiting is passive: You are not in charge, nor are you involved.

One way to counteract the situation is to say, "Well, since you're already interviewing, I'd at least like to be one of the people you interview." Sometimes that little bit of assertiveness may help you get the interview. The only risk involved is that you may spend the time going to the interview only to find that they had pretty much decided on the other candidate. But you may find that they like you better.

Even if you do not get the interview, all may not be lost. At the end of the phone call, after all the platitudes—"Sorry I didn't call you sooner. Thank you for talking with me...."—always add, "Why don't I send you my CV in case something materializes in the future or things don't work out with the physician you're interviewing."

Either way, getting the interview or just sending in your CV, you are seen as being active rather than passive. And even if they do not hire you, they may remember you when their colleagues call to say they are looking for someone in the field. You will have added another link to your network.

NETWORKING

Networking is the best way to find a job. Having a personal referral gives you an edge on other candidates because the decision makers are already biased in your favor. Why? Everyone knows that people will not refer you unless they are almost positive you will be a good candidate and a good fit. When people refer you, their credibility is on the line. They will refer only people who make them look good. So, because they can be fairly sure of a good fit, busy physicians and administrators would rather find one candidate through referral than have to sort through five hundred CVs of people they do not know.

Think about it. What would you rather do—call a few people whose judgment you trust to get names of possible candidates or try to determine possible candidates from hundreds of pieces of paper that tend to look pretty much the same? Say, for example, that you are in a group of noninvasive cardiologists and you want to bring in someone to do invasive work and to set up an invasive cardiology lab at a hospital. You are a physician first, not a recruiter. You hardly have time to do your own work, let alone spend time searching out job candidates. So obviously you are going to tap your own network before you run an ad.

If you have developed your network carefully, if you are "well wired," you may be the candidate who is referred. You may be "discovered." Your chairperson, your attendings, and your peers all have their own networks. And when people in their networks call to ask for names of possible candidates, you want yours to be the one they give.

One resident, for example, was discovered for her job when her chairperson gave her name to someone he had trained with. The chairperson's friend had called looking for "emergency-trained physicians who can think on their feet and who get along well with others." The emergency room at his hospital, an excellent, large regional medical center in a high-density service area in Ohio, was going to be designated as a trauma center. The chairperson told his friend to call the resident: "She is an excellent physician who is respected and liked by everyone she works with. She's usually the calm at the center of the storm in our emergency room. By the way, she's from Cleveland." The friend called the resident, she was interested, she went for an interview, and she got the job. She had no competition at all. And she never even prepared a CV.

Another physician was discovered for his job when he got a telephone call out of the blue from a physician who was looking for a replacement for the otolaryngologist who was retiring from his group. Six months earlier, the resident had heard that a large group was looking for an otolaryngologist who could do plastics. But when he called, he found that the group had just hired someone. He talked for a while with the head of the search committee and, of course, sent his CV as a follow up.

At their annual meeting, the head of the search committee was talking to a colleague who said that his group was looking for someone who could do plastics and that they were getting ready to run an ad. The head of the committee remembered the resident: "I got a call a few months ago from a young man who had heard we were looking for someone. We had already found our candidate, but he impressed me as bright and articulate and was very personable. He also seemed to be well trained. He sent me his CV. When I get back, I'll give you his name and phone number. You might do well to give him a call." He did, and the resident got the job. Not only that, but the job was better suited to the resident: The group was smaller, and the location was better.

One of the best things about being "discovered" is that you are in the catbird seat. You are in a much better position to negotiate. Why? Because the decision makers do not want all the bother of running an ad and weeding out candidates and doing reference checks. They are seeking you out. You are not just one of a number of people being considered for the job. You are their choice.

Being discovered is obviously the most effective and efficient way to get a job. If you are discovered, people will talk about how lucky you are. But finding a job this way is not as passive or as lucky as it seems. Luck is what happens when hard work and opportunity meet. People who lie back and wait for the miracle to happen will probably wait a long time. Discovery is the result of careful preparation—developing excellent clinical and interpersonal skills, building a solid network, searching out opportunity, and making the most of the opportunity when you find it.

RESPONDING TO ADS

Responding to ads, especially to blind ads, is the most common and least productive method of finding a job. It is also the most passive method. And that is one of its problems—the people hiring tend to see you as passive. Not that they do not respect you for responding to their ad—they just do not see you as someone who is out there making things happen.

Another problem with this method of finding a job is that most often the best jobs are not advertised. As you have seen in the section on networking, advertising is the least efficient and effective way of finding someone for a job. Busy people just do not have the time to track down the best candidate through the mountains of letters and CVs that result from an ad.

The number of letters and CVs points to the biggest problem for you with responding to ads—the competition. How many people do you think have responded to the same ads you have? One ad for a general surgeon in the Northeast elicited more than seven hundred and fifty responses. Even if you want to go to an underserved area, the competition will still be intense. A resident finishing training in nephrology in Chicago replied to an ad for a nephrologist in a small town in Idaho because she had grown up nearby and missed the "laid back life out there." She later found that more than one hundred people had answered the same ad.

In both instances, only a few people who responded to the ads were invited in for interviews. Another problem with this method is that you may spend a great deal of time and money answering ads and never hear anything at all. Once you have sent in your CV, you have to sit around and wait for something to happen.

If you do get a response to your application, especially if you have applied to a blind ad, you may find that the job is one that you would not even consider. One resident thought he had found his job: "The ad sounded exactly like the job I'm looking for. When the letter came back, I knew it contained good news because it was thick. Refusal letters, when you even get them, are always *very* thin. I was so excited I didn't even look too carefully at the return address. I called my wife so I could read the letter to her as soon as I opened it. The job was in a city infamous for its fog and the respiratory problems of its population. I have asthma."

The job may be in a location you like, but when you go for the interview, you may find that you do not like the professional environment or even the people you would have to work with. A resident in orthopedic surgery, an Orthodox Jew who had very carefully arranged his interview so he could meet the rabbi and go to the synagogue, thought he had really found his job—all the way through dinner on the second night of his interview. Everyone was so relaxed and happy with each other that over coffee some of the members of the interview committee began telling jokes, racial jokes. He did not take the job: "If they tell jokes about blacks, you can be sure they tell jokes about Jews."

In responding to an ad, you may find a great job. But the unknowns on both sides of the equation make that possibility statistically weaker. For example, both the general surgeon and nephrologist jobs eventually went to referred candidates—because the people hiring *knew* about them. When faced with hundreds of responses, potential employers judge the applicants for the job pretty much on the basis of their credentials, choosing people who went to the best medical schools and trained in the best programs. Yet, as everyone knows, the best credentials do not always guarantee the best candidate. The CV is two-dimensional, a flat piece of paper that says almost nothing about who you are.

Do not, however, discount the importance of your cover letter and your CV as a foot in the door. When asked how they ever made their way through the seven hundred and fifty applications for thegeneral surgeon job, every member, but one, of the search committee admitted having followed a two-part, rapid weeding out process. If the cover letter contained even the slightest error or was sloppy, the application went into the "round file," the equivalent of the trash basket. If the letter was obviously a canned one or if it was "cute," the application went into a "probably not" pile. Said one member of the committee, "You'd be surprised at how quickly it's possible to reduce the number of applications that way. You have to wonder what they're thinking about. One guy even applied for the wrong job."

The next step in the process was to look at the CV, not for content, but for presentation. Again, if it contained any errors, even punctuation errors, it went into the round file. If it was done sloppily or was a poor copy or was done with a dot matrix printer, it went into the round file. Using this process, the committee members reduced the number of applicants to under thirty—in only a couple of hours.

Clients often ask search consultants and recruiters not to help candidates with their CVs because the clients want to see how much time and effort they are willing to put into a seemingly trivial task. One consultant tried to convince a client that although a research associate candidate for a job in his department did not have a good letter or CV, the candidate was really an excellent physician. The client's reply was, "If he's so good, why didn't he prepare a decent cover letter and CV? What does this [the letter and CV he was shoving across the desk] say about his research? See any accuracy or attention to detail in this?" The candidate did not get the job.

If you are going to respond to ads, take the time to write a good cover letter that is neat, accurate, and well written. Make sure your CV is done in standard format (See Figure 5). It, too, should be correct. If you have any gaps in your education or training, fill them in. You do not want people to wonder where you were during those two or three years. One physician had spent two years in Vietnam, but on his CV did not say anything about his military service. Fortunately, when the search committee began to discuss the possible implications—people always assume they are negative—of the missing two years, one of the members who had been in Vietnam himself looked at the dates and guessed where the physician had been.

Your Name, M.D. or D.O.
123 Oak Street
Elmsville, Anystate 00000

Summary of Qualifications
Completion of _____ Residency, June 1987*
Experience in a (Specialty), group-based Urgent Care Center
Emergency Room training and experience
Anystate license
NBME certification
Board Eligible, (Specialty)

Education and Training†
Fellowship: (Specialty), July 1985-June 1986
                   Any Hospital, 456 Any Street, Pines,
                     Anystate 00000
Residency: (Specialty), July 1984-June 1985
                   XYZ Hospital, 78 Fir Street, Appletown,
                     Anotherstate 00000
Internship: (Specialty) or Rotating Internship, July 1983-
                     June 1984
                   PQR Hospital, 6 Cedar Street, Limeburg,
                     Anotherstate 00000
Medical School: Doctor of Medicine or Doctor of
                     Osteopathy May 1983
                   Any Medical College, Kiwi City, Anystate
                     00000
College: Bachelor of Science, Cum Laude, May
                     1979
                   Any University, Anytown, Anystate 00000

Specialty Board Status
Board Eligible (or Board Certified), Governing Body of Specialty

Medical Licensure
State
National Board of Medical Examiners, Certificate, 1986†
ECFMG, FMGEM, FLEX†

Figure 5. Sample CV

(continued on next page)

Professional Experience†
  Title. Name of Organization. 123 Birch Street, Beechtown, Anystate, July 1986-present
  Title. Name of Organization. Address of organization. August 1985-June 1986, approximately forty hours per month
  Title. Name of Organization. Address of organization. September 1985-June 1986, approximately twenty hours per month

Military Service†
  Title. Branch of military. Place, Address. Dates

Honors and Awards†
  Name of honor or award, date awarded

Membership in Professional Organizations
  Name of organization
  Office held, dates†

Research Projects†
  Name of project. Name of director, Director (if any). With Name(s) of colleague(s) (if any). Place. Address. Dates

Publication†
  Use standard bibliographic form. List most recent first.

References
  Supplied upon request

---

* Never abbreviate addresses or dates

† If applicable

Note: Do *not* include personal information such as marital status, age, hobbies, children.

Spend the extra money to have your CV printed professionally—on off-white, eggshell, or oyster heavy bond paper. The *very slight* color difference just may make your application stand out from all the white ones. But, of course, the most professional printing on the best paper will not help if the CV contains errors of any sort.

Responding to ads is not very effective under the best circumstances. At least give yourself a chance of being asked for an interview by making sure every part of your application is done perfectly.

MASS MARKETING

Mass marketing, using direct mail, is another common way of trying to find a job. It is also relatively unproductive. One physician mass marketed herself to every free-standing psychiatric hospital and every acute-care hospital with an inpatient psychiatric unit on the East Coast. She did not get one interview.

The most obvious disadvantage of mass marketing yourself is the small return on your investment of both time and money. Nationally, the average response to mass marketing is around two percent. You may be lucky and get a two percent return. But, just as with responding to ads, you may not be interested in the responses you do get. Again, when you explore further, you may find that the job is in the wrong place. Or you may not like the professional environment or the people you would have to work with.

Another problem is getting your CV to the right person, to the decision maker. If it gets to the wrong person, it may end up in the trash. Or the person who gets your letter may mean well, may mean to take it to the chairperson or the CEO of the hospital. But even if he or she thinks you are an outstanding candidate, he or she may just forget. After all, doctors are busy, and dealing with a potential candidate is not a high priority, unless the group or hospital is in the midst of a search for someone in your field.

Timing is another problem. You really have to hit when people are looking for a candidate. Often people looking for a candidate for a job say, "I got a letter a couple of months ago from someone who sounded very good. But I don't know what I did with it." A search firm ended up placing the psychiatrist who had mass marketed herself all over the East Coast—at a place she had written to. The people there had absolutely no memory of ever getting her letter and CV.

If you do get your letter and CV to the right person at the right time, you can do very well. For one thing, the search committee will see you as active, as someone who tries to make things happen. For another, you might have relatively little competition, especially if you hit at the beginning of the search. Once word gets around that a place is looking, you may have more competition. But at least you will not have as much as you would have had by responding to ads. Again, though, your cover letter and CV have to be excellent. If they are not, you do not stand a chance.

One way you can help your chances is by following up your letters with telephone calls about a week after you think people have received the letters. If you have sent large numbers of letters, making telephone calls may seem an impossible job. But you should try to find the time to call the places you are most interested in. Doing so will make people see you as active, as a go-getter. The call may remind whoever got your letter to take it to the appropriate person. And you will have made another contact.

USING A PLACEMENT FIRM

Using a placement firm is essentially a way of extending your network. A good placement firm can save you much time and money. Why? Instead of marketing yourself, you can have a placement firm do your marketing for you. Involved with nationwide professional placement networks, these firms know of jobs available all over the country. And usually they know of good unadvertised jobs because more and more employers are using placement firms to save themselves time and to make sure they see the best candidates. The result is that many of the good jobs are, in effect, being taken off the market.

Many times physicians avoid using these firms because they think they are employment agencies. They are not. If you go to an employment agency, you pay the agency a fee. If you are accepted as a candidate by a placement agency, the employer pays the fee.

Another reason physicians avoid using placement firms is that they become annoyed by the many calls and letters they receive from the firms. The calls always seem to come at the wrong time—when you are in the hall or on rounds. You are paged, and you go to the telephone only to discover that the caller is a recruiter. So you say, "I'm busy right now. I'll call you back." But you never do. Unless you already have a job or are sure you will have, you might do well to call the recruiters back. One of them just may have the job you are looking for.

As in any profession, some firms are excellent and some are not. The problem is determining how professional a firm is, especially during the first telephone conversation. If you ask the right questions and the recruiter knows about the profession, you will probably establish rapport with the recruiter because you will think the recruiter understands you and the kind of job you are looking for. Some will, but others will really just be talking a good game.

When you find a good recruiter, you have really found an agent, someone to do most of the work of job searching for you. But when you find a bad one, you may be complicating your life. With some, you may send your CV and never hear from them again. Or they may ship your CV to hundreds of places around the country—and you end up getting calls from every small hospital in America. Or they may give you a hard sell, convincing you that an opportunity is so good that you would be a fool not to look at it, even if it does not meet any of your requirements. So you end up job shopping through someone else.

How can you tell the difference between professional and nonprofessional recruiters? One way is to use the first telephone call effectively. Find out how much they do know about the medical profession in general and also about your specialty. Also, find out *specifically* what they can do for you. Have some probing questions ready so you can determine which is which: where is the nearest invasive cardiology lab, how many deliveries per month, has the emergency room been certified as a trauma center, what kind of equipment is available for the procedures you do, what is coverage like, what is the service area?

Another way to tell the difference between a good recruiter and a bad one is to understand the way the different types of placement firms work. Basically, there are three types: "paper houses," contingency search firms, and retainer search firms.

Paper Houses

These are the ones you want to avoid. They buy CVs from sources such as the *AMA Placement Register*. Then they may or, more likely, may not call you before sending your CV out as a piece of direct mail to groups, HMOs, and hospitals all over the country. If by chance one of these places follows up and calls you, the paper house receives a fee. Suddenly you are getting calls from places you would never think of going to, and you become angry. The calls take time away from your work and your patients, and they infringe on the time you should be spending job searching. Do not, however, let your irritation with these firms put you off the good placement firms.

Contingency Search Firms

These firms operate by searching for clients who are looking for physicians and then getting a verbal or written contract which says that if the firm sends a candidate whom the client hires, the client will pay the firm a fee. Sometimes the client pays the fee when you sign your contract, sometimes when you actually begin to work, and sometimes half when you sign and half when you begin.

Once the firm receives the commitment from the client, the recruiters begin searching for candidates to fill the job. Good ones will spend a great deal of time with you on the telephone. (This is a telephone-intensive business.) They will listen carefully to both your personal and professional needs and will try to put you in touch with opportunities that would suit you. If they find that you and the job they are trying to fill are not a good match, they may ask your permission to send your CV to another firm in their network which they think might have a job you would consider.

The term *recruiter* actually covers only part of their job. They spend as much time marketing physicians as they do recruiting them. If they are impressed with you and find you to be a strong candidate, recruiters will actually market you to other firms. One resident wanted to move as far as possible from Seattle because he had just gone through a painful and turbulent divorce. A recruiter in Seattle marketed him to a Maine recruiter who found him a job there. Why did the Seattle recruiter go to all the trouble? She received half the client's fee.

If they find you to be a top candidate, recruiters will market you directly to clients who they think could offer you the kind of job you are looking for, calling them and "selling" you to them. When they find a client who is interested, they get a verbal commitment from the client and then put you in touch with the client.

Or, if they are really impressed by you, they will use you as a primary marketing tool. They will call hospitals, groups, and HMOs in the part of the country you want to go to and ask if they need a plastic surgeon, for example. In the process, the person they talk to may say, "No, we don't need a plastic surgeon right now, but one of our OB/GYNs is retiring and someone in nuclear medicine is leaving. Do you know any good people in those fields?" At that point, if they get a "job order" for those two places, recruiters might put your CV aside while they go to their data base and manual files to see if they have an OB/GYN and a nuclear medicine physician who might be interested in those jobs—because the person at the other end of the line has just agreed to pay them a fee if they can fill those jobs.

However, good recruiters certainly will not abandon you. In the process of recruiting for the two new jobs, they may turn up something for you. Since they are always on the telephone talking to people who want to hire physicians or to other recruiters who want to fill jobs, they hear of new opportunities all the time. Many potential employers who use placement firms would rather work with a half dozen or so contingency firms than pay a retainer search fee and work with only one firm. So recruiters are in touch with many different kinds of medical groups.

The fact that recruiters do most of their work on the telephone points to one of the disadvantages of using a contingency search firm. Recruiters sometimes do not have as much information about a job as you might want. They may not be able to answer all your questions about it. And they may not have a strong professional relationship with the client. Also, they may not know enough about you or your specialty to know if you will be a good fit. They often know neither clients nor candidates personally. As a result, you may end up going to an interview for a job that is all wrong for you, to an interview that is essentially a waste of your time.

But the advantages of using a search firm far outweigh the disadvantages. If you know what you want, if you have done all your preliminary work for deciding on a job, you should be able to assess the quality of both the recruiter and the prospective job. When you find recruiters you can work with, set up parameters with them for the kinds of jobs you will look at and for how or even if you want them to market you.

Retainer Search Firms

Retainer search firms work for their clients. A large multispecialty group, for example, may ask a firm to find an anesthesiologist. And the group will then pay the firm a retainer fee to do the search. Clients use retainer search firms because they want a professional to do all the preliminary screening and prequalifying for them. They are busy doing their own jobs and would rather just be presented with two or three candidates who they are pretty sure would be a good fit than take the time to go through the search process themselves.

Because retainer firms work for the clients, you can be sure that the consultants have a strong and very close professional relationship with the clients. The clients trust the consultants to find them the best candidates. Retainer consultants go to the places they are hiring for, get to know the people involved in the program, finding out what they want and what they are like. So they will be able to tell you everything you want to know about the position.

Retainer firms have three levels of people working on searches—researchers, recruiters, and consultants. The researchers compile a list of names of possible candidates. Often they use the consultants' expertise to help in the process. Because the consultants work so intensively in the health-care field, sometimes concentrating on a single specialty, they have strong networks and know whom to call to get the names of the best residents finishing up each year and of the best physicians with the qualifications the client is looking for.

The researchers give the list of names to the recruiters who do the preliminary screening of candidates. Called *prequalifying the candidate,* this phase of the process is usually brief. Recruiters either write or call first to set up a time for a call in which they ask basic questions to try to determine if you would be a possible candidate for the job. They then give the list of prequalified candidates to the consultants.

The consultants call the candidates to arrange a time for a lengthy phone call, up to one-and-a-half to two hours. In these calls the consultants weed out about ninety-five percent of the prequalified candidates. They try to find out as much as they can about you—and not just about your training and clinical qualifications.

They want to know what you see as an ideal practice opportunity and what you would be willing to trade off on that ideal, your lifestyle and professional and financial priorities, your spouse's occupation, your home town, your spouse's home town, and the ages of your children. When they have put together a picture of you and you seem to be a viable candidate, they will often arrange to fly in to interview you in person and to interview your spouse or significant other too.

They want to recruit your spouse as well as you, because if your spouse is not interested, you are not a viable candidate, no matter how interested you may be. One physician, for example, went to a first interview while his wife was in the hospital having a baby. He loved the job, the people, the place. And he arranged to bring his wife for the second interview—his wife who had told the consultant, "I'll go anywhere that Harry thinks will be a great professional opportunity." When they arrived, his wife would not even get out of the car: "I'd never live here. I hate it here."

If the jobs the consultants describe to you sound interesting, do not do what some physicians do and say, "Why should I deal with you? You're just the intermediary." You not only have to interview with the consultants, but you also need to impress them in the interviews. If you do not, you will never get near those jobs that sound so interesting.

You should treat interviews with consultants exactly the way you would treat job interviews. The consultants are the first line in the interviewing process for the jobs. Dress appropriately and be prepared to answer questions frankly. If you say your chairperson thinks you are a wonderful person when the two of you have a personality clash, the consultants will learn the truth when they do reference checks.

After interviewing potential candidates for a job, usually five to ten, the consultants pick the two or three they think are the best fits and present them to their clients in one of two ways. They may present the candidates all together and have the clients judge them candidate to candidate. Or they may present the candidates as they find them and have the clients judge them candidate to criteria.

Either way, they will arrange an interview for you. They help the clients structure the entire process, making sure that everything runs smoothly, from having someone pick you up at the airport to arranging informal social gatherings so you can get to know the other physicians to setting up a separate itinerary for your spouse. The consultants also prepare you for the interview, making sure that you understand the job you are interviewing for and that you will present yourself in the best light.

Actually, consultants coordinate the entire job search process from your recruitment to your contract signing. They help you negotiate the contract and are there to act as intermediaries, discussing the clients' concerns with you and yours with them. As you move into negotiations, if you do have concerns or problems about the job, tell the consultant so the client can address your concerns.

A married couple, for example, interviewed at a Boston hospital and both were offered jobs. His job was to be only half-time hospital-based practice and the other half private practice. Because he was to be half-time, the hospital was going to pay only half benefits and malpractice insurance. He told the consultant that everything about the job was perfect, that his wife was prepared to accept her job, but that he could not afford even half Massachusetts malpractice insurance. The consultant talked to the hospital administrators who agreed to pay full malpractice insurance for the first two years. Having everything go well is important to the consultants' professional success.

So you can be sure of their help—even on problems that arise a year or so after you take the job and you think you need a mediator.

Another advantage of working through retainer search firms—in addition to the mentoring that you get from consultants—is that you have very little competition for the job. Usually you are competing with no more than one or two other physicians; sometimes you are the only candidate.

One disadvantage is that retainer search firms will not market you. If you are a particularly strong candidate, consultants may give your name, with your permission, to another retainer firm. But most often, if things do not work out, they just put your name in their data base. Another disadvantage is that if for some reason, you want to leave the job in which they placed you, during the first couple of years, the retainer firm cannot work with you. They have agreements with clients that they will not recruit away from the job for a specified time, usually two years, or for as long as they work for the client. But again the advantages outweigh the disadvantages.

One thing to be very careful about as you try to search for the perfect job: Do not become so caught up in the search that you become one of what Ernie Johnson, chairperson of physical medicine and rehabilitation at Ohio State, calls "tire kickers," the people who spend all their time looking for a car by kicking the tires but never get in to drive it. Do not become a job shopper, spending all your time chasing down the elusive perfect job. Remember that neither perfect physicians nor perfect jobs exist.

Chapter VIII

Surviving the Interview

The interview is the final hurdle of the job search. And it is an important one. It is where you see if that job you think is ideal is really for you—or if you are ideal for it. An interview is merely a conversation between two people, but it just happens to be a business conversation.

Before you have a face-to-face interview, you may have a telephone interview. Although the telephone interview is usually just for fact-finding and for setting the date for the *real* interview, treat it seriously. In this interview you begin to establish rapport with one of the decision makers. If the call comes at a bad time for you or if you do not feel prepared to talk about the job, ask to arrange another time for the call. You want to be just as clear and prepared in this type of interview as you are in any other, because preparation is the key to interviewing.

Just as you have planned for every other phase of the job search, you must plan for the interview carefully. If you are nervous about interviewing or if you have not interviewed much, try role-playing with one of your peers. Be tough on each other—ask difficult, probing questions. Do not rehearse the questions ahead of time because you want to be able to gauge your reaction. You do not even need to set up special times—fire surprise questions at each other as you walk down the hall or sit in the cafeteria. Also, be honest with each other about the quality of your answers.

If you cannot find someone to role-play with, do it yourself. Do what one physician recommends: "Try it out on the doorknob." Pretend you are talking to someone out loud. Ask yourself the questions you would ask if you were on the other side of the desk, and answer them. Also, ask the questions you want the interviewers to answer. You will be surprised at how effective role-playing is in reducing interview stress.

You also should do background research on the place where you are interviewing, especially if it is owned by a large corporation. You want to be able to talk intelligently and to ask intelligent questions about the size, diversity, corporate structure, problems. So find out as much as you can. Doing so may save you from the fate of a recent college graduate who interviewed with ICI America. One of ICI's college recruiters has a standard question: "What do you think of foreign-owned business in the U.S.?" The graduate fell right into the hole, saying "America for Americans." Had he prepared for the interview, he would have known that ICI is a British firm—and he might have gotten a job there.

Also, find out as much as you can about the people who will be interviewing you. Try to get your itinerary far enough ahead so you can memorize the names and titles of everyone you will meet. Use your network. Call people who might have trained with your interviewers or who might know them.

One smart move is to do a literature search, especially if you are interviewing with an academic institution. Get copies of the interviewers' articles and books if you can. And while you may not have time to read everything thoroughly, you can at least skim the material. The idea is to get enough information so you can make intelligent remarks about it. People are enormously flattered to hear that other people know about their work.

One other thing that is helpful is to learn, if possible, what the people look like or at least to get a general idea of their appearance. If you can, you will be able to walk toward the people when they meet you at the airport. Even if you cannot, make an educated guess. When you see the people you think are your interviewers, walk toward them, put out your hand, and say, "Hello, I'm Jane Doe. You must be Drs. Smith and Jones." Why should you go to all the trouble? Because going toward people instead of waiting for them to find you makes you appear active and assertive. First impressions matter.

Since shaking hands is one of the first things you will do, remember the advice in Chapter II—"never let them see you sweat." If you tend to have sweaty or cold, icy hands, go into a rest room and run your hands under warm water for a few minutes just before you meet your interviewers. That way your hands will be warm and dry when it is time to shake hands. If you are not prone to sweaty palms but just want to make sure, unobtrusively rub your hands on your skirt or trousers just before you step forward to meet the people.

Another thing, whether you are a man or a woman, is to make sure your handshake is firm—no dead fish and no bone crushers. If you are a man shaking hands with a woman, do not assume she is too delicate for a real handshake. Shake hands with her exactly the way you would with a man. And when you shake hands, look people in the eye and speak clearly and distinctly. Nothing creates a worse impression than people who look away and mumble into their coats.

WHAT TO WEAR

Another component of your first impression is, of course, the way you dress. You must look like a professional, so your dress must be professional—conservative, not loud or flashy. Professional dress gives you an air of quiet confidence, and it inspires confidence in those around you. One or two good interviewing outfits are a good investment in yourself and in your future. Remember that historically physicians have been as conservative as the most conservative business people.

Stories abound of people turned down for jobs because they wore inappropriate dress to the interview. One woman did not get a job she wanted because she wore polyester pants to the interview. One man did not get his job because he wore his "doctor" shoes to the interview. Both these people had excellent credentials; they were, in fact, among the top residents in their fields. When the committee was asked why they were turned down, the response was much the same in both cases: "We want people like us—and they're not. We don't dress that way." A chairperson of internal medicine said, "There's so much in the air these days about how to dress for success and that sort of thing that there's no excuse for someone coming in here in a plastic suit. It's inappropriate behavior, and physicians are supposed to be especially sensitive to inappropriate behavior. I wouldn't hire people who weren't dressed appropriately, not because of their clothes per se but because of what their choice of clothes says about them."

All these things may seem trivial to you. And the idea that you will be judged on them as well as on your ability to practice medicine may seem especially trivial. But you will be. If you are a successful physician, you need to look like one. You have spent too much time studying the effect of the unconscious on people's behavior to ignore it now.

Men

Buy at least one suit of a natural material, probably wool, or of a *high quality* natural-synthetic blend. The most practical suit would be a charcoal gray or navy blue pinstripe. Solid black or navy is too formal. It looks more appropriate for evening wear or funerals. The suit should be single breasted with a single vent in the back. Though very European, the double-vented suit is not generally considered conservative American business attire.

Do not even think of skimping on tailoring. Gaping necks and lapels and jackets, sleeves, and trousers that are too long or too short all shout, "Cheap." The suit neck should drape snugly around your neck, leaving about an inch of shirt collar showing, and the lapels should lie smoothly against your shirt. The jacket length should be just about the same as the sleeve length; the sleeve length, about a half an inch above your wrist; and the pant length, long enough for a slight "break" in the crease. Make sure that everything fits well, with no bagging or stretching of the material.

Your shirt should be long-sleeved, white, one-hundred percent cotton Oxford cloth, with a button-down collar and button cuffs. French cuffs with cuff links may be too flashy; save them for more personal occasions. The shirt should be well pressed and new—lightly starched, with no ring around the collar or frayed collar or cuffs. It too should fit well, with no gaping collars or sleeves that are too long or too short. The cuffs should ride just a little below your wrist bone. Unless your shirt is opaque, remember to wear an undershirt. Having your chest show through your shirt is bad form. Never leave your top collar button behind your tie unbuttoned. Doing so suggests that you are careless.

Your tie should be silk or wool challis. Knit ties are too casual. For the pattern, regimental stripes are safest, but a conservative club or school tie will do. The best color is burgundy with gray or navy stripes or tiny white polka dots. Just remember that tiny is the key word. The knot should be neat and not too large. It should not cover the whole area between your collar points. Length is also important. The tie should reach the top of your belt buckle. You do not want to be remembered as "the guy with the short tie." With a good tie, length should not be a problem. But if you are exceptionally tall, you can buy an extra-long tie, just as you can buy a long shirt.

Shoes are another item that you cannot skimp on. If you are a fairly standard size, you might be able to get away with a medium-priced suit or shirt. But shoes say it all. You could buy the best tailor-made suit available, and ruin everything with cheap shoes. One CEO admitted, "I know it isn't quite humane and all that, but there is a part of me that judges people by their shoes. Shoes that are those plastic clodhoppers or that are scuffed and run-down at the heels make me see the person a little differently." So buy a good pair of black, tie dress shoes. And make sure that they are highly polished and that the heels are new.

Also, invest in a few pairs of very good socks, preferably made of a fine wool or cashmere blend. They should be black or navy, depending on the color of your suit—no argyles or bright colors or, worst of all, white. And they should be at least three-quarter length. You do not want a great expanse of hairy leg showing when you cross your legs.

The look you are aiming for is conservative and understated, especially if you are interviewing in an academic institution or in a metropolitan area. A physician who interviewed to be head of emergency medicine at a teaching hospital in a major East Coast city did not get the job because he wore a tweed jacket and blue shirt with his doctor shoes. The head of the committee said, "Our emergency medical department has just been given a level-one certification as a trauma center. We want the head of it to project a more professional image than Dr. X does."

If you are interviewing in a rural area or in a small community, you may be able to wear a blazer or a tweed jacket and loafers. But even there, everything needs to fit well, to be well made, and to be in good condition. The old days of the rumpled, unkempt physician who is too busy thinking great thoughts to care about appearance are gone.

Obviously, your jewelry should be understated. Leave flashy rings and gold chains at home. If you have to have your gold chains for good luck or whatever, at least keep them hidden. Huge sports watches do not work with pin-striped suits. If you do not have a dress watch and you do not want to buy one, borrow one. Do not wear a tie clasp or pin. And, most especially, do not wear lapel pins of any sort. One candidate lost a job because he wore a lapel pin showing his affiliation with a religious group. An influential board member effected the turndown, not because she objected to his religious affiliation but because she objected to his proclamation of it: "There was no reason for his wearing it. He was here to interview for a job in his profession, not in his religion."

Women

Women have a little more leeway in their dress than men do. You do not have to be a male clone in a skirt instead of trousers. But the same rules apply—be conservative, understated. The most practical thing for interviewing is a good suit in a natural fabric. If you are interviewing in hot weather or in a warm climate, a linen/synthetic blend works better than all linen because it will not wrinkle as much. The safest colors are dark gray, navy blue, or medium blue. Or you can choose a coordinated suit—a patterned jacket with a solid skirt or vice versa. Just remember, if you do, that suits of this sort make you look shorter and sometimes, depending on the style, heavier.

Pick a style that flatters you. The jacket can have a collar or be collarless; it can be short or long. The skirt can be straight, but *not* tight, with a kick pleat. Or it can be flared—plain or with an inverted pleat or pleats. The most important thing is that your suit be well made and well tailored. Go to a store that does tailoring, or take the suit to a good tailor. Just be sure that the hem of the skirt is even and comes just below your knee, that the jacket sleeves come just above your wrist, that the neck and lapels fit smoothly and do not gape, and that the material does not bag or pull anywhere. A minor consideration—replace the buttons if the suit has cheap or gaudy ones.

Shirts, preferably made of silk, should be simple but stylish. Soft, flattering styles and colors work much better than stark white versions of men's shirts, especially when they are combined with one of those silk ties or rosettes that are often touted as "professional looking." You do not want to be remembered as "You know, the woman who was dressed like a man." Choose any color you want as long as it complements your suit and your own coloring. In fact, an interesting color or print or style (as long as it is in good taste) might give you a little individuality.

If for some reason you feel uncomfortable in a suit, you can wear a dress. But it must be a conservative, business dress—no bold or flowery silk prints, no cleavage. The fabric should be wool or a linen blend in a quiet color—again, probably dark gray, navy blue, or medium blue—and perhaps pin-striped. The dress should be well-constructed and tailored, with long sleeves, probably a belt, and a simple straight skirt.

Good shoes are essential. Invest in a pair of fine leather pumps that are fashionable but not extreme. Obviously, you do not want slingbacks or sandals of any sort. Heels should not be exceptionally high and should be in good repair. Make sure the lifts are new, and have a reliable cobbler fix any tears in the heel leather. Your shoes should also be highly polished, or well brushed if they are suede. The color should coordinate with your suit or dress—a dark color is most practical.

To go with your outfit, wear natural or tinted, *sheer* stockings. They can be dark or gray or eggshell or white, even in winter. In summer, stay with lighter colors. Stockings should not be bright or patterned or have seams. Buy more than one pair. You will need backups in case you get a run. And make sure they fit well, with no sags around the ankle or a crotch that comes halfway down your thighs. You need to give all your attention to the interview, not have part of it on the uncomfortable crotch seam rubbing against your legs as you walk.

Also, buy a *good* leather handbag that either matches or coordinates with your shoes. Like cheap shoes, cheap handbags can ruin the effect of your outfit. The bag should be medium sized, large enough to hold the essentials without bulging, but not a huge, cavernous sack.

Keep jewelry to a minimum. Do not wear big, dangling earrings or five gold chains or ropes of pearls. Clanking bracelets are distracting. "Interesting" rings with huge stones, real or otherwise, are too flashy. Sports watches are out. Invest in a dress watch or borrow one. Remember that understatement is the key.

Keep makeup to a minimum, too. You can certainly wear it—probably should wear it—but use natural and subdued colors. Do not wear extremely bright or dark colors. Use blusher, eyeshadow, eye liner, and mascara sparingly. If you are not experienced at applying makeup so it looks as if you are not wearing any, get someone to work with you until you learn how.

One of the problems for female physicians is the way some of their male colleagues treat them—as helpless little girls or as sex objects or both, or, on the other side, as "men." Do not intensify your problems by coming to an interview looking like Alice in Wonderland or Marilyn Monroe or Gertrude Stein. Look like what you are— a successful professional female.

For both men and women a good overcoat is necessary if you are interviewing during cold weather. The coat should be conservative, well tailored, made of wool, and simple in a subdued color. A woman's coat should be long enough to cover her skirt. If you do not want to invest in a woolen coat right now, both men and women can wear a plain street length trenchcoat. Gloves and scarves, if you wear them, should be like everything else—quiet and of the best quality that you can afford.

At this point many of you might be saying what one resident said when a search consultant was advising him about what to wear: "You talk about fashion; you talk about good cut. What do I know about good fashion or good cut? The only good cuts I know about are cuts on people. When have I had the time for this stuff? Or the money?" If you have not had the time, early in your last year of training, take some time to look through fashion magazines to see what is in style. Find out the good stores in your area that serve professional people, and go to them to look at the clothes before you have to buy any for interviewing.

Interviewing outfits will entail a large outlay of money. So if you do not feel sure about your clothes sense, take along a friend who does. Ask the salespeople for suggestions. Often they can be very helpful. Before you buy, go back to the stores two or three times to try on different suits so you can see what looks best on you. When you are finally ready to buy, take the same friend along so he or she can help you make tailoring decisions.

If you really cannot spend a great deal of money, find out about good discount stores. When you have determined what you want to buy, go to one of them. Often you can save a couple of hundred dollars. But you will have to get the tailoring done someplace else. Some areas also have very good discount shoe stores, but here you have to be especially careful not to get outdated styles. The secrets of using discount stores to advantage are to know exactly what you are looking for and to know the difference between well made and shoddy.

Grooming

For both men and women, good grooming is essential. Physicians have to be squeaky clean and neat. Hair should always be freshly washed. If you have dandruff, use dandruff shampoo and carry cellophane tape so you can remove the dandruff from the shoulders of your dark suit. For men, beards and mustaches should be well trimmed and short—nothing outlandish.

Invest in a good haircut. And remember that haircuts look best when they are about a week old. Men's hair should be short, with the ears cut out. Women's hair should also be short and simple—blunt cut or layered, whatever works best for you. If you really want to keep your hair long, go to a good hairdresser to have it neatly trimmed and styled and to have the hairdresser show you how to pull it back from your face when you go on interviews so you'll look more tailored and professional. Also, if your hair is dyed, make sure it looks natural.

Your fingernails should be *clean* and well shaped. Men's fingernails should never come beyond the ends of their fingers. And women's fingernails should not be long, certainly not long enough to cause comment. Long fingernails are not practical for a physician. Although you can wear polish, it should be subdued. For both men and women, a manicure is another good investment.

Unless you are icy cool and completely poised in interviews, do not wear any aftershave, cologne, or perfume. If you feel lost without your signature smell, use only the smallest amount. You will be nervous, and you know what being nervous does to your body temperature. Then your body heat evaporates the alcohol in the cologne or whatever, intensifying the aroma. And the committee walks around all day in your cloud of Polo or Joy—probably not the way you want to be remembered.

Special Problems

What do you do if you look young, if people always assume you are still in school? Dressing conservatively will, of course, make you appear to be older. If you have glasses but usually wear contacts, wear glasses to the interview. If you are a woman and you still have long, straight hair, get it cut and styled.

How can you camouflage extra pounds? Both men and women can wear slightly longer suit jackets. Women can wear a loose jacket over a business dress or a solid color suit with a flared skirt. But the most important thing is to make sure your clothes fit well, with no popping buttons or bulging pockets. Tight clothes make you look much heavier.

What if you perceive your height to be a problem? Usually height is a problem only to the individual, not to the people around him or her. If you think you are too short—usually men, just remember not to strut around trying to overcompensate. Be yourself, and have confidence in what you know and who you are. If you think you are too tall—usually women, do not slump over, hoping to look shorter. You will just look insecure. Women who feel this way should wear a coordinated suit rather than a solid color one, but not flats. They make you look unprofessional, not shorter. The secret in both instances is to have good posture and to move well. If you do not have good posture or if you move awkwardly, practice.

Once you are dressed and ready for the interview, forget about how you look, forget about your clothes. Do not tug at your tie or pull your lapels or fiddle with your skirt. If you are not comfortable in "dress-up clothes," wear them a few times when you are with your friends in nonstressful situations. Make your clothes part of you. If they fit well and you are sure they look good on you, doing so should not be a problem.

Do not play with your hair or constantly brush or toss it back from your face. Do not stroke your beard or fidget with your earrings. Do not put your hands anywhere near your mouth—a sure sign of insecurity. In fact, keep your hands away from your face altogether.

HOW TO MOVE

Your carriage and the way you move and sit say a great deal about the kind of person you are. A woman who interviewed to be an associate medical director did not get the job because, according to the medical director, "she looked like a bag lady in disguise." She was dressed appropriately, but she slumped when she was standing and sitting and shuffled when she walked. She also looked down at the ground most of the time. As the director said, "Everything about her screamed lack of confidence. You can't do this job if you're afraid. You have to project assurance and confidence."

Stand up straight and walk briskly. A quick pace suggests that you are assertive and task oriented. When you are having the hospital tour, move along with the people giving the tour; do not meander along behind them. You can stop to ask questions as you go. In fact, doing so will show that you are active and knowledgeable. Just remember to keep up the pace. The first visit is to give you an overview of the facility. You do not need to see every corner of every department. This is familiar ground to the other people. They are used to walking through these halls quickly.

During the interview itself, sit up straight (but comfortably) and lean slightly into the conversation. Acknowledge what the interviewers are saying by nodding frequently, maintaining good eye contact, and looking receptive, with eyes open and a pleasant, expectant expression. Also, use expressions such as "I see," "yes," "really?" to give verbal acknowledgement. Just remember to vary the expressions. One young physician lost a job opportunity because he irritated the client by saying "okay" after everything that anyone said to him.

If you are a woman, do not be coy. Do not lean your face on your hand, tilting your head to the side and batting your eyelashes. If you are a man, do not be "unbuttoned." Do not lean back in the chair with one foot propped on your knee and your arms swinging over the back of the chair. All these things make the wrong kind of statements about you. A male physician interviewing with a female medical director propped his feet on the desk and pointed his crotch straight at her. Whatever his statement was, he did not get the job.

Maintain good eye contact throughout the interview. You do not need to stare the people down, but you do need to keep looking at them. A psychiatrist with excellent references and training was turned down for a job because he never looked at the interviewers. Even during lunch, he answered questions and asked them with his eyes fixed firmly on his club sandwich. Not looking at people makes them think you have something to hide.

Get your friends to tell you about any nervous habits—gestures or fillers in your conversation—that you might have. And correct them. The repetition of a nervous habit is distracting and irritating. The young physician who constantly said "okay" admitted later that just about a week before the interview one of his fellow residents had told him about the habit—"But I didn't think it was that important." It is. If you can, have yourself videotaped.

You may resist the suggestions in this section because you may think they will make you too self-conscious. So you say, "I am who I am. Love me or leave me." That is a mistake because correcting nervous habits, poor eye contact, and negative body language will not only improve your interactions with interviewers, but doing so will improve your interactions with patients. You will be a better physician as a result.

HOW TO ESTABLISH INITIAL RAPPORT

When you go into the interviewer's office, you are moving into the crucial phase of the interview. Even though everything may have gone well to this point, people often become nervous when the door closes and they are face to face. The important thing to remember is that the interviewer is probably nervous too. The interviewer wants the process to work as much as you do.

Be active. Find something to break the ice. You can mention something interesting or amusing that happened on your way to the interview. Take a quick look around their offices to see what you can learn about the people. They might have photographs of their travels or paintings of the Wild West or stuffed pheasants. Whatever, comment on it, ask about it. If you are not usually aware of the things around you, practice before you begin interviewing. When you go into someone's office, ask yourself what you could use as a conversation opener.

If you have done your literature search and have read something by your interviewer, comment on it, perhaps even ask a question or two about it. Doing so will immediately get the person on your side. You can even talk about the weather. Everyone jokes about using the weather as a topic of conversation, but it is a safe and easy way to phase into the interview.

The beginning of the interview is really just a chance for both of you to get to know each other, to establish some background so that you are at ease when you move into the more complex areas of training and philosophy. To do this, people will often say, "Tell me about yourself." Remember that this is not your cue to begin with "I was born." Your interviewers will be asleep before you even get to medical school.

Focus continuously on the fact that this is a business meeting. You might give them a *brief* background sketch, but try to relate things to your professional life. For example, you might describe how you became interested in medicine when you were a child and watched doctors dealing with a sick grandparent or when you were a teenager and volunteered in a hospital. People will be interested in this kind of information, not in whether you played field hockey or soccer in college. More personal information about your life will come out later, perhaps over dinner or drinks.

Occasionally you might run into some difficulty during this initial stage of the interview. You may return to people's offices with them, only to find that they have stacks of papers on their desks and six phone calls to return. Not everyone is a good interviewer. The person may become abstracted and begin shuffling through the papers rather than focusing on you. Here is your chance to show how sensitive and insightful you are. Say, "It looks as though a lot of work has piled up while you were out of the office. Don't mind me if you need to answer some of your messages. I can certainly amuse myself for a few minutes." The person might say, "Oh no. Nothing is terribly important. Let's talk instead." Or he or she might say, "I really do have to make one or two quick calls," and you can offer to leave the office for a few minutes. Either way, your interviewer will see you as someone who is aware of what is happening around you.

HOW TO LISTEN

One of the things you must discipline yourself to do during the interview process is to listen very carefully to everything people say to you. One of the problems for many people in situations such as interviews is that they have two or three tapes playing in their heads— all at the same time. So while your interviewer is asking you about your experience with a procedure, you may be thinking, "Do I like this person? What would working here be like? I wonder about ..." Or your mind may be racing ahead to questions you want to ask or you think the interviewer might ask you. Turn off those tapes and focus on what the person is saying. You will have plenty of time after the interview to think about the people and the job.

If you do not understand a question, use reflective listening. Say, "Excuse me, but did I understand you correctly? Are you asking about my interest in ICU or my experience in ICU?" In doing so, you will have accomplished two things. One, you have given the interviewer time to clarify the question, perhaps to ask a better question. Two, you have given yourself time to think about how you want to answer that question. Actually, you have accomplished a third thing: You have let the interviewer see that you are a good listener.

Another thing you should do is watch your interviewers' facial expressions and gestures as you answer questions. Pick up cues from them. Do they look puzzled? Try to find out why. Do they fidget? Cut short your answer. Do they seem irritated? Try another tack. The point is to try to answer their questions as clearly and succinctly as possible.

The worst thing you can do is take a shot at what you think the interviewers have asked and end up not really answering the question. They will remember you as someone who is vague, as someone who avoided direct answers. You want them to remember you as someone who is incisive and to the point.

HOW TO BE ACTIVE RATHER THAN PASSIVE

As you get to the heart of the interview, your goal is to be active rather than passive. Do not sit languidly answering the thousand questions your interviewers fire at you. Take just as active a part in this conversation as you would in any other. To be active, of course, you have to be prepared. You have to have information not only to answer questions but also to ask them. You have to have thought about the kinds of questions you might be asked. Look at an interview as if it were a giant puzzle. If the interview is successful, all the pieces will fit in the puzzle. By the time you leave, the interviewers see you not only as someone who can do the job but also as someone they would like to have do the job because you understand it.

Early in the interview you should ask them to tell you the daily responsibilities of the position. Say you are interviewing to be a new cardiologist in a group. As your interviewers describe what they would expect of you and what procedures you would be expected to perform, you can describe your experience in each of the areas.

Another good question to ask early in the interview is one about the philosophy of the group or unit. So, for example, if you are interviewing to be an allergist in a multi-specialty group and the interviewers tell you that they take a holistic approach to patient care, that they see patients' families as extensions of the patients and their problems, you can tell them about your experiences in working with families and about your interest in the whole patient.

You can ask them what kinds of problems they see in the practice. They may say that they are losing some patients to a new group because the group has an assertive, energetic business manager who gets referrals through networking and marketing to other hospitals in the area. If you are energetic and entrepreneurial yourself, you can tell them some of your ideas that might counteract the loss of patients.

The idea here is that you are letting them see specifically that you are a good fit, that you fit into the puzzle of their organization. After you leave, they will not have to sit down and discuss point by point whether you can do the job. By the time they have shaken your hand at the end of the interview, they will know you can do the job.

Another good reason for asking these questions early on is that good interviewers ask open-ended questions that give you an opportunity to expand on your background, training, and interests. Knowing what they are looking for helps you structure your answers so they can see you can do the job. Remember that you do not want to leave them with questions about you.

Other questions you might ask are ones about how the group or hospital operates: Do you have any HMO or PPO contacts? What is the role of a junior partner? How many patients do you see each day? What kinds of procedures do you do? How many of each type do you do? What kind of equipment is available for complex procedures? Would you be willing to add equipment? In an academic institution, is the position tenure track or not; what is the ratio of research to teaching time; what is the role of an instructor or of an associate professor? Questions such as these show the interviewers that you are prepared, interested, and knowledgeable.

You can be active rather than passive in answering as well as in asking questions. One question, for example, that people will be sure to ask you is "What are your weaknesses?" Instead of answering, "I'm weak in laser surgery," turn your answer around so it is more positive: "Although I haven't had as much opportunity as I'd like to do laser surgery, I hope that when I begin to practice, I'll have more opportunity to get experience in this area."

If they ask you about personal weaknesses, you can again state your answer positively. And remember that a personal weakness, one that may interfere with your personal life, may be a professional strength. So if you are compulsive about your work—if you are still at the hospital at 8:30 p.m. checking on patients or if you stop by to check on a patient when you are on the way home from the Y after working out—you can say, "Well, my spouse complains that I'm a workaholic. I seem to have a difficult time leaving my work behind." If you genuinely cannot think of a weakness, you might say, "I'm sure I have many weaknesses that my spouse could tell you about, but I really can't think of any offhand that would interfere with my work." However, if your weakness is that you are always late, correct the weakness before you begin interviewing.

Another question you will probably be asked is "What are your strengths?" This is not the time for false modesty. Knowing your strengths is just as important as knowing your weaknesses. Discuss your strengths as objectively and rationally as you would any other topic. The idea is to let the interviewers see that you understand who you are.

You may be asked "What was the worst experience you had during residency? How did you handle it?" Tell them about the experience. They were residents, too, and had their own worst experience. You can even turn the question around and ask them about their worst experiences—a good way to establish camaraderie. They may ask "What was the most difficult case you've ever had? How did you handle it? What was its outcome?" Again, discuss the case openly and honestly. And ask them what kinds of difficult cases they get, what kinds of difficult cases you might expect to see if you work with them. Every time you ask them questions of this sort, you are helping to establish yourself as part of the group, you are fitting yourself firmly into their puzzle—the last piece that will make everything complete.

People will frequently ask you questions which might be somewhat difficult to answer: What would your peers say about you? How do you measure up to the other residents in your year? What would your chairperson say about you? Answer each of these as honestly and objectively as you can. Your interviewers will appreciate your spontaneity and candor.

Remember that people tend to hire people they like. One way to make sure your interviewers will like you is to be open during the interview process, to share your experiences freely, both good and bad.

HOW TO DEAL WITH DIFFICULT SITUATIONS

Occasionally in an interview you will run into difficult or awkward situations. Everyone has either experienced or heard stories about stepping in the ice bucket or watching two of the interviewers go after each other. The thing to do when these sorts of things happen is to try to turn them to your advantage. If you step in the ice bucket, stay poised and make a joke at your own expense. If you are in the middle of two people working out old grudges, say something tactful about many opinions about that procedure and change the subject. Remember that doctors constantly have to deal with difficult situations. If you show in the interview that you can, you are one step ahead.

Sometimes you will be asked a question that you really have no idea how to answer. Do not answer it just to give an answer. You will seem stupid. That is a good time to say, "You know, I'd like to give that a little more thought because I'm not sure about it. Could we come back to it later?" But be sure to come back to it later. At the end of the interview, you could say, "Now that I've had a little time to think about that earlier question, I think I'd do this" or whatever. If you still have no idea, say, "I still don't feel as if I could answer your earlier question without giving it some additional thought."

Again, your interviewers will see you as someone who is open and honest. No one expects you to be perfect.

Sometimes, in trying to be honest with you, your interviewers may give you information that you will find difficult to respond to, that you will feel awkward about. When this happens, try to reflect the speaker's feelings. So if the interviewer tells you that the group's best physician just died of a heart attack at the age of 35, you do not need to say anything profound, just something to show you understand: "That must have been very sad," or "That must have been a terrible shock." Or if the interviewer tells you that the group has had to let someone go recently because the other physicians were not happy with his or her patient care, you can say, "That must have been difficult. What were some of the problems?" Although none of these responses would show your intelligence, they would show your empathy. You will have other chances to demonstrate your intelligence. And good doctors are empathetic.

Some of your interviews will be well structured, with each member of the committee focusing on different areas of your background and experience. But others—and these are the most difficult—will be set up so that you are meeting ten different people in half-hour slots, and all ten people will ask you the same sorts of questions. By the time you finish with the fourth or fifth person, you will be tired and a little shell-shocked from having to answer the same questions over and over again.

The problem for you here is to keep up your energy and enthusiasm throughout the day. If you do not, you will begin to project an ennui and lack of interest that you do not intend. Remember what is at stake, and concentrate on listening carefully and on projecting energy and enthusiasm.

Another problem is that you will probably forget what you have said to whom, whether you asked this question to the physician you are talking to now or to the one you talked to three hours ago. Be honest and approach the problems openly: "Excuse me, I don't want to be redundant. But I've met so many people today that I can't remember if I asked you this question earlier." You'll impress them with your honesty and interest—and you'll help them understand your difficulty in the interview.

Although these are difficult interviews, you can help yourself out a bit by taking some control of the situation. If someone asks you a question you have answered three times already, you can answer briefly and say, "I've talked about these things with a number of the other physicians. But I do have a couple of things I'd like to know more about." Then ask some of the questions you have thought about while you were preparing for the interview: What are the long-term goals of the group? Where do you see yourselves as a group in five years? Do you plan to take on PPO contracts? Asking these questions will help you refocus the interview and will help keep your interest up.

Meals are often difficult for people. The thing to remember is to order something that is easy to eat. If you do not feel too secure with a knife and fork, do not order Cornish game hens. Order something that will leave you plenty of time to concentrate on the conversation. Unless you grew up on the Chesapeake Bay, do not order steamed crabs. Make life easy for yourself in a situation as stressful as this by knowing in advance approximately what you will order: lunch, salad or club sandwich; dinner, fish or meat.

You are there to talk, not to eat. Order the same type of food everyone else is having. Unless you have strict dietary rules, reading the menu from cover to cover and being finicky about the wine are bad form. You want to impress your interviewers as a physician, not as a gourmet or a gourmand. You certainly do not want to do what one hungry young physician did—order two entrees. Deciding quickly on something you feel comfortable eating will allow you to concentrate on the issues. And because you will feel at ease, your interviewers will see you as someone who is poised and in control.

If you are staying overnight, especially if you are with your spouse, you may be asked to a cocktail or dinner party. Do not be lulled by the social atmosphere; this is a difficult situation. Your social, interpersonal skills are constantly being measured. People are asking themselves, "Is this someone I want to associate with day in and day out?" If you are rather shy or introverted, make an effort to be more extroverted. Smile, shake hands, ask people questions about themselves. Remember that the people hiring are looking for someone with good soft skills, someone who can establish quick rapport and understanding.

Another hazard in these social situations is the "bombers," people who are threatened by your coming into the group or the area. Bombers are likely to corner you and say, "You know, Jane (or John), I really like you, and I'm telling you this because I don't want to see you starve. But you just won't have the patient base here to make a living." Thank them politely, but never take their word. Check out their information *before* you leave, especially before you write off the job.

A few years ago, for example, a small community hospital that had a number of internists was bringing in its first noninvasive cardiologist. During the formal interviews everyone was very polite and encouraging. But during a dinner party that evening, four or five internists took him aside—one at a time—to tell him how much they liked him and how little he would make.

Although he had made a verbal commitment to the president of the hospital, he left town the next day and called another place where he had interviewed to tell them he had changed his mind and was now interested. The search consultant tracked him down in a hotel where he was about to sign another contract; the hospital president, hearing what had happened, asked each of the internists to call him to reassure him. He accepted the job and five years later is practicing successfully in the community. So watch for the bombers.

WHAT NOT TO DO

Do not bring up the subject of money, especially at the beginning of the interview. Money is not discussed until the end of the first interview or even until the second. You can, during your wrap-up interview or on the ride back to the airport, very tactfully ask, "Could you tell me a little about your compensation and benefits package?" Asking this sort of question at the end of the day will say to your interviewers that money is not your most important criterion in deciding on the job. People do not want to hire people who are interested mainly in what they can get.

Do not become so comfortable during the interview that you begin telling lots of jokes. That does not mean that you cannot laugh or tell about some funny things that have happened to you. Humor can be an excellent ice breaker or tension breaker—when used with caution. But many jokes have racial or ethnic or sexist or sexual overtones, even when they are not explicit, so you are bound to offend somebody. And some people just cannot stand jokes, with the inevitability of the stupid punch line and having to laugh at it. Save your comedy routine for friends. The interview is a business conversation.

HOW TO LEAVE

At the end of the interview, maintain the assertiveness that you have had through the rest of the interview. If you are interested in the job, say so and ask, "Where do we go from here? What's the next step?" The worst thing is to get on the plane not knowing whether you are to call them or they are to call you.

Also, try to establish a time frame. Find out when they expect to make a decision. If you have a time frame for deciding about your options, let them know it. That way you can try to reach a mutually convenient time for them to let you know their decision. They may not be able to let you know in time. But at least you will have let them know you have other offers. If they want you, they will get to you before your deadline.

Occasionally you will be offered a job on the spot. Many people feel they need to be cool and not to appear too eager. Or they feel foolish if they accept right away. One physician called the search consultant from the airport, giggling and almost hyperventilating. When she asked what was the matter, he said, "I think I've done a terrible thing. I just accepted the job. I know they'll think I'm overanxious, but it's just what I want. I talked to my wife last night on the phone, and she liked the sound of it. So when they offered, I said yes." Accepting that job was not a terrible mistake. If everything feels right and the job meets your personal, professional, and financial needs, take it.

If you do not, you may end up like the young physician who after the interview knew he really wanted the job. But because he thought he should not seem too eager, he said, "Well, I am interested. I'd like some time to think it over, though." He waited about a week and a half before calling back and finding that the group had already hired someone else whom they liked just as much. When you find a job you want, do not play games. The market is too competitive. No law says you cannot accept a job at the end of the first interview.

What if you are not really sure about the job at the end of the interview? Remember that in the interview process chemistry is just as important as content. When you are back home, try to picture yourself in your white coat, mingling with those physicians every day, walking down those hospital corridors, operating in that operating room, seeing patients in that office. If you can see yourself there comfortably, the chemistry was probably good—for both you and the interviewers. They will probably be able to see you in the job also.

But what happens if everything does not click in the interview? You will have gained valuable experience and information that will help make your next interview better. Interviewing is a learned process for some people. Look at an unsuccessful interview as a learning experience. A bumper sticker says, "Experience is what you get when you don't get what you want." The important thing is to learn from the experience—and not to be discouraged.

THE SECOND INTERVIEW

If everything does click, you will be called back for a second interview. The second interview means that the people hiring are serious about you as a candidate. And your accepting the second interview should mean that you are serious about the job. Job shoppers, who string everyone along in their quest for the perfect job or the best offer, are often left holding an empty bag at the end of the process. Somehow people are able to sense that you are not a serious candidate, so they hire someone else. They become irritated that you have wasted their time. News travels through the network that you are a job shopper, and you end up with nothing. Do not go back for a second interview unless you are almost positive that you want the job and will accept it if it is offered.

If you do go back, try to arrange to bring your spouse or significant other along. Ideally, your spouse should go on the first interview, but having him or her come to the second is practically a necessity because the search committee will have arranged for you to meet a relocation specialist. Relocation specialists are experts on the area. By talking to you and your spouse to get an idea of your special needs, they steer you to the right neighborhoods for you. They explain the cultural, educational, and recreational opportunities available. In effect, they sell you the area.

The second interview is also the time you will probably visit schools to see if they meet your children's or spouse's needs. Your spouse might use this time to explore job opportunities for him- or herself. You will most likely meet the spouses of your colleagues. What you will actually be doing is getting an overview of what life will be like for you if you take the job. You can see that coming to a firm decision about the job would be difficult, if not impossible, if your spouse does not accompany you.

Just make sure that your spouse stays in the background during professional interactions. For example, having your spouse sit in on salary and benefit negotiation is perfectly acceptable. Even asking an occasional question is all right. But the spouse should be there primarily to listen. One spouse lost a job for his wife because he had a list of things to discuss and kept interrupting and negotiating for her. The committee decided against her: "If she's so good why does she need her husband to negotiate for her? What will she do in difficult situations when he's not there to tell her what to say?"

Another spouse did much the same sort of thing. Interviewing for an academic position, the physician was asked to give a lecture. In the question-and-answer session afterward, his spouse kept interrupting and answering questions for him. Again, the committee decided not to hire him: "Whose research was it? What will he do when she's not there to tell him what to say?"

As well as exploring what the job will mean to you personally, you will be exploring it even further professionally. This is the time to make sure you understand absolutely what the job is. What is the group's philosophy about patient care? What would your specific role be in the group? What kind of coverage is available? What kind of research time and space will you have? Are they willing to add equipment that you need for your research or procedures? How much CME time will you have? What kind of growth are they predicting? Without this kind of information you will not be able to make the best decision for you.

During the second interview, you will probably discuss compensation and benefits. (For a more detailed discussion of negotiating contracts, see Chapter IX.) Very often you will be asked what it would take to get you there. So be prepared. You should have figured out your lowest acceptable offer. Do not, however, quote that; quote what you would like. If, for example, you know that people in your specialty in that geographic area are starting out with a base around $85,000, you can say that you would like to have a base somewhere around $100,000 for the first year but that the figure is negotiable. And negotiate from there.

Occasionally, if the negotiations are complicated, you may be asked back for a third interview. This interview is really just an extension of the second. You may meet more people and see more of the area. And you will fine tune the details of the contract. Whatever the particulars of the third interview, if you get to it, you will have survived the interview process.

Chapter IX

Getting the Offer and Negotiating the Contract

During the second interview you should be actively striving for an offer. And at the end of the interview, make sure that what you have is a bona fide offer. Often people negotiating for their first jobs confuse the intent of the people hiring. Over and over again candidates tell search consultants that they have an offer, only to discover that the decision maker is just an "interested party." You need to know the differences between an interested party, a verbal commitment, a letter of intent, and a contract.

An interested party is just that—someone who is strongly interested in you but for whatever reason is not ready to make an offer. A verbal commitment, on the other hand, means that both of you are saying yes: Yes, the job is yours; yes, I will take the job. The verbal commitment is a tentative acceptance; it does not tie you to the job. If all goes well and it looks as if you can work out the details of the job, by the time you leave the second or third interview, what both you and your interviewers will probably be looking for is a verbal commitment, something that will allow you both to stop searching and get on with negotiating an acceptable contract.

A letter of intent often follows the verbal commitment. More binding than a verbal commitment, a letter of intent locks both of you into the job until the details are spelled out in the contract. It is in many ways the first draft of the contract, often giving both of you a chance to see if either has misunderstood any part of the agreement. You may, for example, see that your two half days each week for your research are not mentioned. So after calling and clarifying your research time, you can pencil in the details, or you can mention them in your cover letter. Either way, they are set out clearly and can be written into the final contract, which nullifies all other agreements between you and the people hiring you.

You do need a contract. Even if you are so excited about the job

153

that you, like one young physician, follow up the verbal commitment with a letter saying, "I overwhelmingly accept this wonderful offer," make sure you get a contract. As one department head said, "Many people just coming out of residency are terribly naive. They just don't seem to understand that medicine is becoming just as much a corporate jungle as, say, investment banking. They shake hands on a job without really being sure about what they're agreeing to. Then in a year they discover they've given away the ranch. There are people out there who chew young docs up, spit them out after a year or two, and then find a new sucker."

One cardiologist, for example, took his first job on a handshake and the promise that "if all goes well during the first year and we find that we suit, I'll make you a partner." The young doctor worked hard, covering five nights a week, and had no problems with office staff or patients. His perception at the end of the first year was that things had gone very well indeed. His would-be partner, however, said, "I don't think things between us have worked out well at all." The young doctor was back to where he had been when he finished his residency, only now he did not have a good reference from his employer. In the course of his new job search, the cardiologist not only found a job in a nearby community but also found that he was the third doctor in three years whom the older cardiologist had used in this way.

Some physicians do not start out to use you, but because they have unrealistic expectations about what adding someone to the practice will mean, they try to alter the original terms of the agreement. Usually when physicians' practices have grown to about one and a half times the number of patients they can comfortably deal with, the physicians bring in an associate. And often they expect that they will continue to earn the same amount of money for half the work. They forget that until the associate brings his or her share of the practice up to a full patient load, some of their former income is going to the new associate. So you need to think ahead for the occasional employer who does not. Get a contract with all the terms spelled out clearly.

The more clearly defined the terms of your job, the more likely you are to have a satisfying experience on the job. You will be able to do your job instead of having to deal constantly with questions about things such as terms of payment, research time, office support, CME time. The better the contract the less likely you are to have to use it. A physiatrist, who has been at his second job for about a year, said, "I didn't know what I was doing when I took my first job. We were always haggling over little things like who was supposed to do the billing. I had just assumed that the hospital would do it all. Now my contract has *everything* in black and white. And I haven't even had to look at it since I got here."

One question that many people going into their first job ask is "How long should the contract be for?" For people just coming out of residency, a one-year contract is usually best. Many people do not stay at their first job. However, circumstances on both sides may make a one-year contract impractical. If you are going to be moving a great distance, for example, you may want a three-year contract so you will not have to deal with all the problems of resettling within a year or two. Or, if the search was difficult, your employers may want a three-year contract so they will not have to deal with the problems of a new search right away.

The same physiatrist, for example, agreed to a three-year contract for his present job because the hospital wants to build the department of physical medicine and rehabilitation so felt it needed some continuity in the chairmanship. Often people compromise with a three-year contract that is renegotiable every year.

At this stage of your career, you probably do not need an attorney to negotiate your contract for you, at least not in the initial stages of negotiation. But, especially if it is complicated, having an attorney look over the contract is a good idea. Even though some employers are using contracts that are written in simple English, that (as one attorney put it) "eschew arcane legalese," many contracts are still difficult for a layperson to read.

In addition to the problem of understanding "arcane legalese" is the fact that some words have different connotations in law than they do in medicine. For example, the word *deny* is a neutral, fairly common term in medicine but a strong one in the law. In doing a review of a patient's symptoms, when you say a patient "denies" chest pain, you mean merely that the patient says there is none. An attorney, however, would interpret your statement to mean that the patient is adamant about not having chest pain. So get an attorney to explain the contract. You want to know *exactly* what you are agreeing to.

SALARY

When negotiating a contract, most people think first of salary. And obviously salary is important. The irony is, though, that you may negotiate a great salary only to find that little things loom much larger when you actually get into the job. Do not stake everything on your salary. An orthopedic surgeon recruited to a city in the south thought he had a great contract, especially a great salary. But he left after a year: "I had one of the best compensation packages of anyone in my year. The problem was I couldn't get anything typed. Reports, histories, everything just piled up. Sure, that was just a sign of lack of support in lots of areas. But that's what I focused on."

Straight Salary versus Guarantee

In negotiating your salary, you should understand the difference between a straight salary and a guarantee and between a net guarantee and a gross guarantee. A *straight salary* is a flat amount of money that you earn per year. Occasionally, you will be offered a straight salary with a percentage bonus of anything over a certain amount that you or your department or your group or your HMO either brings in or does not spend. If you are going to be hospital based or to work for a staff-model HMO, you will probably receive a straight salary. Some large groups also pay a straight salary for the first year.

Most often you will be offered a minimum guarantee. A hospital or group or even a solo practitioner bringing in a potential partner will guarantee that you will make a certain amount of money for the first year, or sometimes for the first two years. In effect, the guarantee is an interest-free loan or cash advance to help you get started. You need a guarantee at first because you will not generate much actual income when you start up your practice. (See Figure 6 for an example of a net guarantee.)

One important consideration for beginning physicians is whether the guarantee is based on billings or on collections. When you are building a practice, a guarantee based on collections is preferable.

The intent of the guarantee is to attract a physician to town at no financial risk. The doctor sets up practice, and the hospital underwrites the doctor's start-up efforts by providing a guarantee of so much net income per year. Net income equals money in, or collections, minus money out, or expenses. Expenses include all costs necessary for the doctor to be in practice, such as malpractice insurance, office supplies, salaries, car expense, rent, equipment, phones, accounting costs.

For example, the hospital agrees to guarantee the doctor $60,000 net income per year, or $5,000 net income per month. If the doctor's net income is less than $5,000 per month, the hospital will make up the difference. If the doctor earns more than $5,000 per month, the surplus is used to pay back the hospital. The following table shows how a net guarantee works.

	Money In	Money Out	Net Income	Hospital Supplement	Net Income to Doctor
January	1,500	3,500	(2,000)	7,000	5,000
February	2,500	3,500	(1,000)	6,000	5,000
March	5,500	3,500	2,000	3,000	5,000
April	7,500	3,500	4,000	1,000	5,000
May	8,500	3,500	5,000	-0-	5,000
June	10,500	3,500	7,000	(2,000)	5,000
July	10,000	3,500	7,000	(2,000)	5,000
August	12,500	3,500	9,000	(4,000)	5,000
September	12,500	3,500	9,000	(4,000)	5,000
October	13,500	3,500	10,000	(5,000)	5,000
November	14,500	3,500	11,000	-0-	11,000
December	15,500	3,500	12,000	-0-	12,000
Total	119,000	42,000	77,000	-0-	77,000

Source: Robert Templin, Roblin Associates, Wilmington, Delaware.

Figure 6. Example of Net Guarantee

Collections can take up to ninety or more days, and the time lengthens as the government gets slower and slower in paying. If, for example, your guarantee is $72,000 and you have collected only $2,000 in the first month, you will receive a $4,000 advance for that month. If the same guarantee is based on billings and you have billed $4,000 but collected $2,000, you will receive only a $2,000 advance for that month. The guarantee based on collections is usually called a *net guarantee;* the one on billings, a *gross guarantee.*

Another drawback to the gross guarantee is that often you will be responsible for overhead. And overhead averages about thirty-five to forty percent of gross income. So try to negotiate a net guarantee, especially if you are joining a developing practice. If you cannot, at least find out the collection rate and the average overhead for your specialty so you will have a general idea of your income for the year.

Other things that you need to be aware of are the schedule of payment—how often you receive the advance, monthly or quarterly—and the payback arrangement. About ninety-eight percent of all contracts require that you pay back the cash advances as soon as your income begins to exceed the minimum guarantee.

Say, for example, that you have a net guarantee paid monthly. In the first six months you receive $36,000 but collect $20,000, and in the last six months you receive $36,000 but collect $48,000. As soon as your monthly income goes above $6,000, you begin paying back the cash advance of $16,000 until you make it up. If in the last six months you produce $68,000, you pay back the $16,000 cash advance from the first six months. But what happens to that extra $12,000?

If you produce more than the guarantee, you will most likely receive all the extra money. But you need to be sure. Sometimes you will receive only a percentage of it. If you do receive a percentage, find out if the percentage is based on gross billings or on net revenues. Many hospitals are moving away from percentages because they require complicated accounting procedures and also because gross sometimes encourages unnecessary tests and procedures and net sometimes encourages underuse of tests and procedures.

PARTNERSHIP OR OWNERSHIP

You need to determine how you become a partner, or owner. Is partnership automatic after so many years? Do you buy in through "sweat equity," or do you actually have to buy in? How much will becoming a partner cost? How will the payment schedule be worked out? How soon can you begin to buy in?

If you are joining a group or partnership, your employers might count everything above the guarantee as sweat equity to buy you into the group or partnership. For example, a plastic surgeon whose practice has grown too large for him to handle alone hired someone just coming out of residency to work with him in his practice. He guaranteed her $100,000 per year for the first two years and is keeping everything above the guarantee as her sweat equity. If she generates the income he expects her to, after two years she will be a full partner in the practice without actually having to buy in.

PROFIT SHARING

Also, if you are joining a group, especially a large multispecialty one, you should ask about profit sharing. Will you be profit sharing right away? Probably not. In one year or two years? Then, you need to determine how profits are shared. Some groups divide all profits equally. Others divide profits by specialty or productivity. So, for example, the surgeons, who usually generate more income, receive a proportionally greater share of the profits. Other groups give everyone the same basic amount and then a percentage by specialty or productivity above the base.

PRODUCTIVITY

If your salary or your percentage above your minimum guarantee is based on productivity, find out how productivity is evaluated. Most groups decide just on economics. If the group does and you are interested in doing other things, such as research or marketing, you will be doing these things essentially on your own time.

Some groups have complicated evaluation procedures—counting things such as research time, CME, and public relations work toward productivity. They may have a special category for administrative work. If the group does have many criteria for evaluating productivity, find out how they are weighed.

ACCOUNTS RECEIVABLE

Another important consideration is when you begin to get a share of accounts receivable. Accounts receivable—money billed but not collected—is often a large part of a group's assets, as much as $40,000 or $50,000 per physician. Usually beginning physicians do not receive any share of the accounts receivable but after the first year may begin receiving an incremental percentage each year. By their fifth year, they will probably be receiving one-hundred percent.

BENEFITS

Many young physicians often forget about benefits when they negotiate their contracts. A good benefits package can add significantly to your compensation. However, as one resident said, "I can't eat benefits." Determine just how important different benefits are to you. For example, you may be offered term life insurance that is double your salary. And that amount may sound enormous to you. Just remember that the insurance would probably cost your employers only about $200 per year. So do not trade off something else for it.

Insurance

One of the biggest questions for physicians is "Who pays malpractice insurance?" Almost always your employers will pay it, but you need to be sure. Depending on the state and your specialty, malpractice insurance could cost you anywhere from $2,000 to $200,000 per year.

Along with malpractice insurance, you should find out who pays the "tail" if you leave. *Tail insurance* is a policy that covers you after you leave a practice for any suits brought against you for something that happened while you were there. Claims-made insurance covers you only while you are actually in the practice. So even though you have malpractice insurance in your new practice, that insurance will not cover suits coming out of your old practice. Tail insurance, too, is very expensive—usually twice your premium for your last year in practice.

Life and health insurance are also negotiable items. Life insurance is usually a term policy that is in effect only while you are employed in the practice. Health insurance, however, can be complicated. You need to find out if your employers pay all or part of the insurance, if the policy covers only you or includes your family, if it includes major medical benefits, and if it is offered through a prepaid plan or through a traditional fee-for-service plan.

Disability

Disability insurance can be quite complicated, so find out exactly how it works. Some policies say that you are covered only if you cannot work, not if you cannot work as a physician. One hospital-based physician discovered that she was not covered as long as she could do anything else—even wash dishes. If much of your income is dependent on your doing procedures, you may want to have a policy that goes into effect if you can no longer do those procedures. One surgeon in an academic setting, for example, has disability insurance that covers him if he can no longer perform surgery, even though he may still be able to teach and do research. Policies of this sort are, however, very expensive.

Another important thing to look into is how long you are covered if you become disabled. Some contracts are void after sixty or ninety days if you cannot fulfill the terms of your contract. So if you have a clause of this sort in your contract, you would not be able to collect your disability after that time. Some disability coverage does not even go into effect for sixty days, so you might not be able to collect at all.

Time Off

Giving physicians time off is very expensive for employers. When you are not there, no one is generating income. Time off includes vacation time, maternity leave for both sexes, personal days, time for attending conferences or seminars, and, in some instances, time for research.

All these things need to be spelled out carefully. Exactly how many days do you get for vacation? Do those days include holidays or weekends? How much time do you get for maternity leave? Is the leave completely full time or will you be expected to work part time during part of the leave? Will you receive full pay and benefits during the entire leave? How many personal days do you get? How are they defined? How are days off for CME counted—as vacation days, as personal days? Or do you get a certain number of days each year specifically for CME? Through all your time off, who is responsible for coverage?

If your job is not research oriented but you want some time for research, you may want to negotiate specific research time. Some employers will give you a full day or two half days each week for your own research; others, only a half day per week.

Retirement Plans

Another important benefit can be your retirement plan. Do your employers have one? What kind is it—an IRA, Keogh, a special plan set up through the group or hospital? Do your employers pay all or only part of the yearly contribution to the plan? If you have to pay a portion of it, how much? Does their contribution depend on yours? So, for example, if you can choose to contribute fifteen or twenty percent, do your employers pay the same amount no matter which choice you make? This is an important consideration for young physicians because you may not want to spend as much of your income on a retirement plan now as you will later.

Other Expenses

A number of other expenses can be negotiated. Such things as relocation expenses, CME expenses, professional dues and membership expenses, parking and automobile expenses, financial and legal counseling expenses, and practice marketing and advertising expenses are often covered by employers, either in full or in part. Sometimes employers also provide mortgage assistance and no-interest or low-interest loans. Or they will help you get them through a local bank.

Practice Support

Practice support is another important negotiable item. You need to determine exactly what kind of support and how much you will get before you sign the contract. Remember that before you sign, you have all the power, so negotiate such things as office space and equipment in advance. Once you get to the job you will be competing with everyone else for money and space. And you will have to wait until the next budget year to try to get what you want.

Practice support includes a number of variables. Do you get office space? If so, how much? Will you be expected to pay for it? Who pays for a practice management consultant if you need one? Do your employers provide furniture and decorating for the office? Will you get support for hiring office staff? For recruiting staff? Do you get billing and transcription support? How are ancillary services provided? You can see that having these things spelled out in advance will greatly simplify your job.

A special consideration is equipment and supplies. If you need certain equipment or instruments for your research or your procedures, employers will usually buy it. But make sure. Do not leave something as important as special equipment or instruments to chance, to "Well, I thought that was understood." Often it is not. An ophthalmologist who neglected to negotiate equipment for specialized laser surgery spent most of her first weeks in her new group trying to get it. She finally did. But she wasted valuable time which she could have spent building her practice, and relations with her colleagues were immediately strained.

PERSONAL CONSIDERATIONS

Have your specific duties and responsibilities defined in your contract. Will you have to spend a certain amount of time doing administrative work and budgeting? Who sets the fees? Will you be expected to do patient management, case management, program management, team management? If so, how much time will be allotted for it? Will you be involved in public relations or practice marketing? If so, how much time will you be expected to spend on it? Will the length of time you spend with patients be monitored? If so, how much time are you allowed per patient?

What kinds of privileges will you have? Sometimes other doctors on the staff will be anxious to protect their own territory, or they may be jealous of your competency. So they may not want you to do certain procedures. If you are in family medicine, for example, will you be able to perform deliveries? You need to make sure that you do not become the group's or department's "gofer." If you are a surgeon, for example, will you get any interesting cases or just the appendectomies?

In modern medicine, peer review is becoming increasingly important. How do your employers handle peer review? How often does it occur? How, specifically, does it affect the terms of your employment? Will you be expected to participate in reviews of your colleagues?

BREAKING THE CONTRACT

Be very clear about what happens if either of you decides to break the contract. Such things as having to pay back guarantees or loans, getting your share of accounts receivable or of your sweat equity or buy-in equity, or being able to set up another practice in the area can vary depending on who breaks the contract.

In general, you will not have to pay back guarantees or loans. If you leave before the end of the contract, most employers just write off the guarantee as a loss. They may, however, renegotiate your loans so you are paying the going interest rate.

Accounts receivable and equity can be difficult items. You need to define the exact percentage you are entitled to. If you leave, you will probably have to forfeit your share of accounts receivable and your sweat equity. You should, however, get back all your buy-in equity. If you are asked to leave, you should make sure that you get your share of accounts receivable. Remember that your share of accounts receivable could be $40,000 or $50,000. Also, you may want to negotiate how the money is paid to you. You will probably want to get it back in yearly installments. If you take a lump sum, you will have to pay heavy taxes on it.

Almost all contracts contain what is called a *restrictive covenant* or *non-compete* clause to protect the practice. This kind of agreement prevents your leaving the practice to set up another one in the same area and taking part of the patient base with you. Make sure that yours is reasonable. It should restrict you for no longer than six to nine months and for no more than twenty-five to fifty miles. When she read over her contract with a large nationwide HMO, one physician discovered that if she left the HMO she would not be allowed to practice within one-hundred miles of *any* HMO owned by the corporation. Her chances of practicing in almost any metropolitan area in the country would have been virtually eliminated. So she hired an attorney who specializes in medical law and renegotiated the contract. Also, the agreement should become void if you are asked to leave. The cardiologist, for example, who "didn't suit" after one year of slave labor was unable to set up his own practice in the community.

Probably the most important aspect in contract negotiations is for both sides to make reasonable agreements. Neither should agree to things that would be virtually impossible to fulfill. Can you really do the specific job you are agreeing to? Can the hospital or group really provide all the things it has promised? Will it be able to pay what it has promised? In your enthusiasm, do not overcommit.

One thing to keep in mind in your contract negotiations is that a well written contract ensures understanding only. Because everything is worked out in advance, you can get on with your job. But it cannot make your job work. Only you can do that.

Chapter X

Setting Up and Managing Your Practice

If you decide to go into a solo private practice which you will have to set up and manage, you will be taking on a complex job. You are probably entrepreneurial and enjoy the challenges of developing your own practice and of running a small business. Be sure to give yourself enough time—at least six to nine months. When you open your doors to your first patients, you must look established. You are not in business until then. Just as in other stages of your medical career, you need to plan this stage carefully. In fact, planning is the key to a successful start-up of a new practice. It is preventive medicine. (See Figure 7 for a checklist of many of the things you must do before you open your practice.)

Each specialty has unique requirements not only for equipment and supplies but also for office layout and design and technical staff. And each physician has special needs. While you are still in residency, try to spend as much time as you can working in the offices of physicians in your specialty. Pay close attention to what works best for you so you can plan your space so that it is more efficient and effective. Also observe the office procedures that seem to make the office run smoothly and the ones that tend to disrupt the office. Spending time in other physicians' offices will help you get some idea of how you want to set up your own office.

Try to attend a practice management seminar. They are offered throughout the year all over the country by the AMA and by consulting firms. Also, special sessions on practice management are sometimes offered at the annual meetings of some of the specialties.

Even if you have been recruited by the community hospital, which has promised to help you start up, you should begin the start-up process by retaining professional advisers: an attorney, an accountant, and ideally a practice management consultant. Your attorney and accountant should have had experience in the medical field. You need

Initial action	Date to Initiate Action	Follow-up Date	Date to Complete
Apply for Medical Licensure	_____	_____	_____
Apply for Hospital Privileges	_____	_____	_____
Practice location			
Find office space	_____	_____	_____
Office layout	_____	_____	_____
Negotiate lease	_____	_____	_____
Sign lease	_____	_____	_____
Equipment			
Order office equipment	_____	_____	_____
Order medical equipment	_____	_____	_____
Order medical sundries	_____	_____	_____
Order filing system	_____	_____	_____
Order typewriter	_____	_____	_____
Order dictation equipment	_____	_____	_____
Order photo copier	_____	_____	_____
Financing			
Apply for loans	_____	_____	_____
Apply for home mortgage	_____	_____	_____
Open checking account	_____	_____	_____
Obtain accountant	_____	_____	_____
Legal			
Obtain lawyer	_____	_____	_____
Important documents			
Apply for BC/BS	_____	_____	_____
Apply for medicare number	_____	_____	_____
Apply for medicaid number	_____	_____	_____
Apply for employer I. D. number	_____	_____	_____
Apply for DEA number	_____	_____	_____
Apply for medical society membership	_____	_____	_____
Telephones			
Obtain telephone service	_____	_____	_____
Install phone	_____	_____	_____
Contact answering service	_____	_____	_____
Place yellow page ad	_____	_____	_____
Order paging unit	_____	_____	_____

Figure 7. Control Sheet for Setting Up a New Practice

Initial action	Date to Initiate Action	Follow-up Date	Date to Complete
Billing system			
Order billing system	_____	_____	_____
Order accounts payable system (optional)	_____	_____	_____
Determine fee schedule	_____	_____	_____
Staffing			
Advertise for employee	_____	_____	_____
Interview employee	_____	_____	_____
Hire employee	_____	_____	_____
Business forms			
Order script pads	_____	_____	_____
Order appointment cards	_____	_____	_____
Order business cards	_____	_____	_____
Order letterhead, envelopes	_____	_____	_____
Patient record forms	_____	_____	_____
Insurance	_____	_____	_____
Obtain malpractice insurance	_____	_____	_____
Obtain office liability and content insurance	_____	_____	_____
Obtain worker's comp.	_____	_____	_____
Obtain personal medical	_____	_____	_____
Obtain personal disability	_____	_____	_____
Obtain personal life	_____	_____	_____
Laboratory			
Arrange laboratory services	_____	_____	_____
Other			
Pick up office supplies & office accessories	_____	_____	_____
Prepare announcement for newspaper	_____	_____	_____
Arrange for pharmaceutical supplies	_____	_____	_____

Source: Thomas Battles, Garofolo, Curtiss & Company, Boston, Massachusetts.

(Figure 7 *continued*)

the attorney initially to review your contract if you have one and later to help you negotiate your lease or mortgage terms. The attorney can also help you decide whether to incorporate. You need the accountant because solo practices are small businesses, and most physicians, especially those developing a practice, have neither the time nor the expertise to run a business completely on their own. Your accountant can help you draw up an initial projected budget and then help you follow it. (See Figures 8 and 9 for typical practice expenses.) Your accountant can also serve as your financial advisor. You also could use the help of a practice management consultant. Management consultants can help you in every phase of your start-up, from designing office space to evaluating your office staff.

Few beginning physicians just decide to go into a community and set up solo practice without the sponsorship of an established physician or of a community hospital. If, however, you have decided to do so, you definitely should find a good management consultant who will help you do a demographic survey or evaluation so you can determine whether setting up a practice in that area is feasible. Even if you are going in with sponsorship, you should ask to see a demographic survey. Look at a number of different factors:

- Hospitals: number and types, possibility of getting admitting privileges, incentive plans (if any) for new physicians in the community

- Physicians: number in your specialty and their ages and board status, number of possible referring physicians

- Population: size, average age, and income

- Major employers: types and type of medical insurance they provide

- HMOs, IPAs, PPOs: types and possibility of participating in them

Also try to find out any unusual patient preferences. You may think, for example, that opening an OB/GYN practice in one city is not feasible because a city only fifteen minutes away has a number of OB/GYNs. But because traditionally patients may not go to that city for medical treatment, you would have a patient base. Conversely, you may decide not to open your practice in a place that already

Medical equipment
   Capital goods   _____
   Supplies   _____

Office equipment
   Furniture   _____
   Typewriter   _____
   Filing system equipment   _____
   Filing equipment supplies   _____
   Dictation equipment   _____
   Photo copier   _____
   Computer   _____
   Decorating   _____
   Initial office supplies   _____

Lease holder improvements   _____

Telephone installation   _____

Billing system   _____

Malpractice (prepaid)   _____

License and permits   _____

Professional fees   _____

Miscellaneous   _____

Source: Thomas Battles, *Garofolo, Curtiss, & Company*, Boston, MA.

Figure 8. Practice Start-Up Expenses

has two or three OB/GYNs. But because they do not like these physicians, patients may be driving twenty-five miles for OB/GYN care. Again, you would have a patient base.

Investigate the attitudes of established physicians in the community to newcomers whom they may perceive as threats to their patient bases. If you are a rheumatologist, for example, the internists and family medicine specialists may not at first be willing to refer pa-

	Monthly	Yearly
Salaries		
Nurse	_____	_____
Receptionist	_____	_____
Education	_____	_____
Benefits	_____	_____
Employee taxes	_____	_____
Rent/mortgage	_____	_____
Utilities		
Electricity	_____	_____
Heat	_____	_____
Maintenance	_____	_____
Telephone		
Monthly service	_____	_____
Answering service	_____	_____
Paging unit	_____	_____
Billing system	_____	_____
Office supplies	_____	_____
Postage	_____	_____
Medical supplies	_____	_____
Drugs	_____	_____
X-Ray service	_____	_____
Lab fees	_____	_____
Insurance		
Malpractice	_____	_____
Office	_____	_____
Worker's compensation	_____	_____

Figure 9. Practice Proforma

	Monthly	Yearly
Health		
Professional fees		
Lawyer		
Accountant		
Management consultant		
Conventions/CME		
Dues		
Journals and books		
Education		
Automobile		
Debt service		

Source: Thomas Battles, *Garofolo, Curtiss, & Company,* Boston, MA.

(Figure 9 *continued*)

tients to you. Doing an evaluation of this sort will give you a much clearer picture of how your practice can fit into the community.

PRELIMINARY PAPERWORK

When you decide where you will practice, apply for state licensure immediately. On average, licensing takes two to three months, but in some states it can take up to a year. Licensing is important not only because you cannot practice without a license but also because a lot of other important documentation depends on your having a license. For example, you must have a license before you can apply for your provider numbers for Medicare and Medicaid. You need these numbers so you can be reimbursed when you treat patients covered under these plans.

You should also apply for hospital admitting privileges right away because sometimes credentialing can be a lengthy process. Most hospitals now require either board certification or board eligibility, with certification within a certain time—usually five years. So you should be on the certification track because in some specialties getting the necessary experience can take a while. For example, if you are an OB/GYN, developing a sufficient surgical caseload will take time.

Also, you have to be able to document your experience in the privileges you are applying for, so keeping good records during your residency is important. If, for example, your specialty is family medicine and you are applying for OB privileges, you have to be able to show exactly how many deliveries you have performed. And think through the privileges you are applying for. If you are the same family medicine specialist, at most hospitals you would not receive GYN surgical privileges. So do not waste time applying for privileges that you know in advance you probably will not get.

You should be applying for other things as well. Once you are licensed, you have to apply for your provider numbers. If you did not receive a Drug Enforcement Administration (DEA) number during residency, you have to apply for one. And, even if you do have a DEA number, you have to fill out a change of address form. Also, check to see the requirements of the state you are going to practice in. Some require the number plus state registration to dispense controlled medications. Although you do not have to, you should apply for membership in the county and state medical societies. They represent physicians' interests at those levels and provide a tap into the referral network.

OFFICE SPACE

At the same time that you are doing all this paperwork, you should be looking for an office. Try to avoid having your office at home, especially if you are just starting out. Patients will see you as available and will just drop by. When you are trying to build your practice, you may have trouble turning them away. The result would be that you would never leave work.

If you are lucky, the hospital bringing you in will have office space available. In fact, many hospitals do marketing surveys and, if they identify a need, build a medical office building or convert space in the hospital to offices. And they then recruit physicians to fill the need and the space. If the hospital does not have available office space, the people there may be able to help you find space in a medical arts building in the hospital service area. Or, failing that, they may be able to identify a realtor who understands both the market and physicians' needs.

Sometimes in choosing office space, young physicians tend to look primarily at cost per square foot. While you must certainly consider comparative cost, other factors such as location and room for expansion are equally important. The cheapest space may not be the best space. You may end up losing money because patients cannot get to your office easily or because you will incur moving expenses when your practice outgrows your space.

If you do find space in a medical office building, you will be in a location already perceived by the community as a place to go for medical treatment. Also, depending on the specialties of the other physicians, you may have an initial built-in referral base. Try to determine the reputations of the other physicians in the building. You may be identified by association with them. Also, if the other physicians are not the owners, talk to them about the advantages and disadvantages of practicing there.

If you do not find space in a medical office building, be careful to choose a good location. Your office should be clearly visible and be easily accessible to your patients, especially your handicapped patients. Parking is important so make sure you have enough space to take care of all the patients you might be seeing at one time. If sufficient parking is not available, check to see how good the public transportation system is. Also, if the office is on the second floor, the building should have elevators, and they should be large enough so that patients in wheelchairs can use them easily.

You also have to think about proximity to the hospital—not only how far away but also the traffic patterns. How quickly could you get to the hospital at rush hour? For some specialties, such as dermatology, proximity is not a major problem; for others, such as OB/GYN, it is.

Some physicians like the idea of converting an old house to office space. Unless you are a psychiatrist and do not need examining or procedure rooms, old houses make good medical offices only if you have a great deal of money to invest in restoration and conversion and plenty of time to oversee the work. General business office space is also not usually appropriate for medical offices and has to be converted.

What happens if you find a place that meets all your requirements but does have to be converted? It can be done. A practice management consultant helped one client to convert a vacant supermarket into a medical office building and another to convert a gas station. Before you begin, check the zoning and building codes to make sure you will be allowed to do what you want with the space. One physician bought a house and had the conversion underway when the neighborhood association met in protest, cited obscure zoning regulations, and forced him out of the neighborhood. Check with people in the area to help you identify a good architectural firm and a good contractor. If you will be working from a distance during the conversion, you will need a liaison, someone on the spot who can deal with problems as they arise, another good reason for retaining a practice management consultant.

If you are leasing space rather than buying, determine who will pay for what and who will own what at the end of the lease. In some states, for example, anything that you affix to a wall, ceiling, or floor—such as lighting fixtures or sinks—automatically belongs to the owner. The landlord might pay for the leaseholder improvements and then factor the cost into your rent. If you pay, you need to determine how the improvements will affect the amount of your lease.

Obviously, you need an attorney to advise you during these negotiations. In addition to who pays for leaseholder improvements and how the payment affects the terms of the lease, you will be negotiating the length of the lease—usually the longer the lease, the lower the rate. Also, moving is costly. You not only have to pay for the actual move, but you also have to pay for announcements to your patients, buying all new business forms, and having a new telephone system installed. And some of your patients may find following you to your new location inconvenient.

When you negotiate the lease, set out exactly what things each of you will be responsible for. The fewer gray areas in your agreement, the fewer problems that you will have to work out once you are there. Small matters, such as who is responsible for cutting the grass, can cause large problems.

In deciding whether to lease or buy, you should get advice from an accountant. Buying sometimes offers more tax benefits and gives you the opportunity to make a good investment. In addition to the potential increase in the value of the property itself, if your space is large enough, you might be able to lease space to another physician under a shared-expense arrangement.

Whether you lease or buy, but especially if you buy, have the hospital help you identify a good bank *and* banker. Or shop for them yourself. Many offer exceptional unadvertised services to physicians only. You will need the banker as an ally, as someone who can provide access to the financial resources you will require. As you set up your practice, you will need lines of credit and mortgage money, both residential and commercial. Because most bankers want to establish relationships with physicians, they are generally willing to lend you money. Even though physicians' overall income growth has slowed, physicians on average still earn more than other professionals.

Plan the interior of your office carefully. Try to use foresight. Many young physicians start with too small an area. Remember that you will need more storage space as your practice grows and that you will need a larger business office as well. If you scrimp now, your office will become more and more inefficient, and you will end up spending more money because you will have to move, expand, or renovate.

Before you begin designing the space, determine how many examining rooms you will need. Most physicians need at least two, but again each specialty has particular needs. Specialties such as family medicine and OB/GYN really need three—one for the patient preparing to be examined, one for the patient being examined, and one for the patient dressing after the examination. A pediatrician usually needs more—an area for well-baby examinations, and one for sick-baby examinations. But the rooms can be smaller. Having enough examining rooms is important because it allows you to move from one room to another efficiently, without having to wait for the room to be prepared.

If possible, try to have one or two additional rooms where your medical assistants can do such things as change dressings and give injections. And try to have a "nurses' station"—a place to review charts before examinations, to make chart entries, to receive and make routine telephone calls. Also consider how capital-intensive your practice is. If you are an otolaryngologist or an ophthalmologist, having more than two rooms with all the equipment you need would be cost prohibitive. When you are starting out, you might have one room with equipment and then a few general examining rooms.

Examining rooms should be approximately eight by ten feet. Anything smaller begins to seem cramped. But, again, you need to decide how you want to use them. A procedure room for casting, for example, may need to be larger; one for EKGs, smaller. Check the way the doors open. Most open against the wall, exposing the room to view, but for patient privacy you want the doors to block the view. Also for patient privacy, make sure the rooms are sufficiently sound-proof that you cannot hear from one room to another. Since most sound travels not through walls but through doors, try to get good, solid core doors. If you cannot, try to deaden the sound by using some form of covering, such as carpeting, on the backs of the doors. Every examining room should have a sink and storage space.

In designing space, try to be as efficient as possible. Have all entrances to examining rooms off a single corridor to reduce time and walking distance. Place sinks and toilets back to back wherever possible to save on plumbing expenses. Be aware of patient flow, and try to design the space accordingly. Also, make sure your corridors are wide enough to accommodate walkers, wheelchairs, and people assisting patients.

Try to provide a space behind the business office area that your staff can use for confidential calls and business discussions with patients. If you are leasing, especially, use as much modular equipment as you can so you can take it with you if you move.

SERVICES AND PROCEDURES

You also have to determine what kinds of services you will offer and what kinds of procedures you will do—for one reason, so you can plan your electrical needs. X-ray machines, for example, require heavier electrical lines than ordinary equipment. Providing x-ray and laboratory services as a convenience for patients is a good marketing device. Patients often become annoyed when they go to their physician only to be told to go somewhere else for an x-ray and then come back. But the cost of providing these services can be prohibitive. If you want to offer x-ray services, you need a room with all interior walls that have lead shielding—an expensive construction cost. If you want to offer lab services such as blood work, you may find competing with the low cost of high-volume labs difficult. Also, for any basic lab work such as urinalysis, you must be able to provide quality assurance.

You must be careful about services and procedures because you do not want to be seen as competing with the hospital. Sometimes you can joint venture, but you will need professional advice to help you determine potential tax problems and the mode of joint venturing that would be best for you.

If you do not provide these services on site, remember to make arrangements to have them done somewhere else. Talk to people at the hospital to see what is available The hospital may provide the services or may be able to refer you to reputable firms that do. If you have to choose your own, find the one that everyone else uses. Other physicians have probably chosen it because it is good.

If you are in a medical office owned by the hospital, you may be allowed to use only certain equipment or laboratory services and be able to do only certain procedures. When you are negotiating for the space, clarify these issues so you will not have any costly surprises once you begin practicing.

BUSINESS OFFICE DESIGN AND EQUIPMENT

Remember that you are running a business. Because this space is the heart of your business, you need to give it special attention. In planning the business office, a practice management consultant is invaluable. Because the consultant knows the local market, he or she can help you identify the vendors with the best service. In choosing electronic equipment, for example, the product itself may not be as important as the quality of service offered in your area on the particular product.

If you can, build in the work area in the business office. If you cannot, get a *good* desk and a *good* chair. A cheap desk is inefficient. The drawers could stick, and it might not have well organized storage space. A good posturepedic chair that has been orthopedically designed may cost more, but you will get more productivity from your office manager. Also, make sure it has a stable base, preferably with five-prongs.

You need a typewriter, transcription machines, calculator, and copier. The typewriter should be the best electronic model you can afford—again, you will increase productivity. The copier should be a plain-bond copy machine for better presentation. The quality level will be determined by how you are going to use it, by the volume of copying you have to do. But, again, remember that although a higher quality machine may cost more, it will increase productivity.

Whether to get a computer is a matter of some controversy. Some accountants say computers are not cost effective. Others say they provide better, more efficient financial controls of billings and accounts receivable. A practice management consultant could help you analyze your practice to see if a computer would be a smart investment. The consultant could also identify a medical computer specialist to help you choose the system and the software that would be best for your practice.

Even if you store records on a computer, you need a filing system to hold hard copies that you can use when you are seeing patients. Only one system is really effective—the color-coded one. This system uses colored bars on the side of each chart, and they are arranged either alphabetically or numerically. The great advantage of this system is that it provides quick resourcing—if a file is out of place, its bar will be a different color from those around it. To store files, you can use either open shelves or cabinets. Open shelves are more efficient, but cabinets are more aesthetic and provide greater confidentiality, keeping the records from the janitorial staff, for example.

As far as the records themselves are concerned, you will probably be most comfortable using the charting system you used in residency. If you are choosing a charting system now, the problem-oriented record is probably the most effective.

COMMUNICATION EQUIPMENT

Telephones are extremely important. They are your tool to do business. Get them as soon as possible. You need your number before you can order many of your business forms. You need to place an ad in the Yellow Pages as quickly as you can. Otherwise you may have to wait for almost a year to use this important source of advertising. You also need good telephones. If they do not work, you do not do business. Go to a reputable firm with high quality equipment and service.

Your answering service is also important. It, like the telephones, is a business-making tool. It is an extension of your office. Some hospitals provide answering services. If yours does not, identify the best service in your area and meet with a representative. Define exactly what you want from the service—what kind of protocol, how emergency calls are to be handled.

Try to coordinate the answering service with the telephones. You will need them at least a month in advance, if not earlier. With both in place, you can arrange to have the answering service book patients for you so you have them waiting when you open your practice.

You also need a good paging service, one with the widest possible coverage and best service. Decide if you want just a beep or a voice or a display. Paging services are often tied into answering services. So check with your answering service and with the hospital. If the hospital provides the service, you will probably get better service for less money.

FEES AND BILLINGS

You must establish a fee profile, usually by talking with other physicians in your specialty in the area. Or you can determine your fee profile from Medicare and Medicaid percentages. However you determine the profile, *never* come in with the lowest fees in the community. You are reimbursed by your fee profile, so if you start low, you will never catch up. Try to raise your fees at least once every year. Often raising them every 6 months in smaller increments is better psychologically. The increments may not be large enough to annoy your patients. Always raise fees in consultation with your accountant. And remember that if you are in a contractual arrangement with a third-party payer such as an IPA or a PPO, the third-party reimbursement will not necessarily change.

Because pilferage and embezzlement are major issues in small businesses such as medical practices, you need a good billing system. Among the best is the pegboard. It is easy to use and inexpensive. It does not, however, give an accurate picture of accounts receivable, and occasionally the ledger cards get lost or misplaced, throwing everything out of balance. Depending on the size of your practice, a more effective way of doing billings might be to have your own in-house computerized system

You can also use a firm that provides billing service. Usually you pay these firms a percentage of collectibles. Pay on gross receipts, not on gross billings. If you pay on gross billings, you will be paying on money you may not collect. Some of these firms just charge a flat fee. The important consideration for you, however, is not the way they charge but how good they are. An ineffective billing firm can cost you a lot of money.

As you begin practice, you may be billing only twice a month, for example, A's through M's at mid-month, N's through Z's at the end of the month. But as your practice grows, you should begin billing every day: A's one day, B's and C's the next, and so on. Billing every day will improve your cash flow. An even better way to improve cash flow, however, is to collect at the time of the visit if the patient is not covered by Medicare or Medicaid or is not in a prepaid plan. Check your accounts receivable monthly, and find a good collection agency for long-overdue accounts. Also make sure that you are charging for occasionally overlooked services such as hospital visits and consults.

Check the state laws for contractual allowances. Some states, such as Massachusetts, do not allow balance billing. So if you charge $100 for a procedure and Medicare allows only $75, you are out $25. Also, if you participate in a capitated plan, find out its collection policy criteria.

WAITING ROOM FURNITURE AND DECORATION

In designing your waiting room, remember that a visit to a physician is almost always anxiety producing. So try to make your office as warm and inviting as you can—and as tasteful. Do not have one of those sliding glass panels between the waiting room and the rest of the office unless confidentiality is absolutely essential and you have no other way of guaranteeing it. Have your office staff wear street clothes rather than white uniforms. The nurse can wear a white coat over his or her regular clothes, just as you do. Choose earth tones because they are warmer than blues and greens. If you are in pediatrics, however, you might want to use primary colors. Use incandescent lighting rather than harsh overhead lights.

Avoid "airport furniture" and imitation leather. For one thing, they are cold; for another, they are almost always cheap. You should buy the best furniture that you can afford. In the end, cheap furniture will cost you twice as much money plus a great deal of time. Go to an office furniture store to get *contract* rather than residential furniture. Contract furniture is made to stand up to wear and abuse. Also, make sure the furniture will be comfortable for everyone. A good fabric covering is usually the best, unless you can afford real leather. You should sit in the chairs yourself to make sure they are comfortable.

Couches are usually not a good investment. They end up being a very expensive single seat. Make sure you have seating space for at least twice as many patients as you ordinarily schedule during peak hours. Also, have at least one or two chairs without arms for obese patients. Use tables and lamps. If you have children in your practice, provide small chairs, a play table, and books and toys. Do not scrimp in the waiting room. It is often your patients' first impression of you.

Pick reading material that is appropriate to your practice. Do not order magazines that reflect just your interests. One physician, a rheumatologist who plays squash and sailboards, has three magazines in her office: one about squash, one about sailboarding, and *Fortune.* Her patients mostly sit and stare gloomily at each other. Also, make sure that your selection is not too affluent, unless you have an affluent patient base. The small-town physician who has *Town & Country, Gourmet,* and *Architectural Digest* also has many disgruntled patients. And keep the reading material updated. You may even want to consider adding a television set.

Personalize your office space. Use your own photographs or your favorite pictures or decoys or old quilts or flowers, whatever. Doing so ties you and your practice together more closely. It helps your patients see who you are. If you use plants, also use a plant service, unless you or one of your office staff is interested in plants and will maintain them. Dead or dying plants do *not* project the correct image.

Keep the waiting room neat. Few things create a worse impression than a waiting room with dog-eared copies of magazines lying around, chairs askew, and bits of paper on the floor.

The same general rules apply for your consulting office as they do for the waiting room. In addition to your desk and chair and a couple of chairs in front of your desk, try to have two or three "soft" chairs grouped around a table. Talking with patients without a huge desk between you is much friendlier and can often be more effective.

A word of advice about business-office, consulting-office, and waiting-room furniture and equipment: getting it can take twelve to sixteen weeks. So order early.

EQUIPMENT AND SUPPLIES

For the business office, you need to order letterhead paper, envelopes, and bill forms; for yourself, prescription pads and business cards. Go to a reputable local printer for these. You also need all the usual stationery supplies. But do not order great quantities of any of these at first. Order minimum amounts, and see how much you use. The same is true for disposables such as table paper, disposable gloves, and tongue depressors. Start slowly until you get some idea of how much or how many you use. Check to see if your hospital sets up special accounts with physicians' offices so you can take advantage of volume discounts.

When ordering your equipment, go to a good medical supply house. Usually these firms will help you define the equipment you need. For example, if you do not know or if you have forgotten that you need resuscitating equipment if you do any kind of injections, they will remind you. They will often lend you equipment such as scopes and autoclaves for short trial periods. Also, they often have their own in-house design staff to help you design your office space.

Take a conservative approach to ordering medical equipment. Make sure that you will use it. For expensive equipment, you might want to consider leasing until you find out how often you use it. If you do use the equipment, you would probably be better off buying it. Again, check with your accountant and banker about the possibility of low-interest financing.

Most physicians do not keep many drugs in their offices. Since you will not need large quantities of drugs, try to work out an arrangement with a local pharmacy or with the hospital. Remember that you will get some free samples from pharmaceutical sales representatives. They also often provide excellent, free educational materials for both your staff and your patients.

INSURANCE AND RETIREMENT PLANS

Another important person in your professional life will be your insurance representative. Get help in identifying the best firm in the area—not necessarily the cheapest but the one with the best service. If you cannot get malpractice insurance through the hospital, the representative will work with you in trying to find the best malpractice coverage for you. In considering the coverage, look closely at the procedures you are applying for. If you do only two or three of a particular procedure each year, you may collect only $300 or $400. But because you may have to pay out $2000 or $3000 in malpractice, you may want to reconsider applying for the procedure. You also need life insurance, personal medical insurance, and disability insurance that will cover you if you cannot *practice*, not if you just cannot work, or you may end up doing dishes somewhere.

For your employees, you need worker's compensation. Check with the governing body of your specialty and with the state medical society to see if they have group rates available. For your office, you need liability and content insurance. You may want to consider office disruption insurance to cover fees you would lose if for some reason, such as a broken water pipe or loss of electricity, you are unable to practice in your office for more than two or three days.

OFFICE STAFF

One of the major overhead items for physicians is personnel. The best place to begin looking for staff is the hospital personnel office. Personnel people either will know of people in the area who are looking or will have resumes on file. If they do not know anyone, check with the local medical society or a placement firm. Advertising is tricky because it can make you look as though you are trying to steal staff from your future colleagues. So you might create a hostile environment before you even arrive in the community.

The key person among the staff is the person working the front office. Usually when you are starting up a practice, this person doubles as receptionist and office business manager. Because this person is so important, try to find someone with experience. Test his or her technical and clerical skills. And check references! This person has access to almost everything you own—on average, physicians generate $200,000 to $300,000 a year—and he or she represents you to the public. So do not hire anyone because of "such a nice face." Also, see if the person will agree to be bonded. Bonding is, essentially, taking out an insurance policy on the employee. Then, if he or she embezzles, you get your money and the insurance company gets to prosecute.

This employee should have good telephone skills and be personable, honest, and discreet. He or she cannot be a gossip or a busybody. Also, the person should have good mathematical and clerical skills. He or she should be able to type from a dictaphone, be familiar with medical terms, and be able to type fifty to sixty words per minute. Fewer than that could cause problems because of lack of productivity. The person should be somewhat flexible—able to work one evening a week and one Saturday a month, perhaps. (Having evening and Saturday hours is an excellent marketing tool.)

Pay this person well. This is one instance where you will absolutely get what you pay for. If you are not sure of the going rate (which you should top), check with the hospital personnel office. Try to hire him or her at least two months before you open your practice so you can have your practice organized when you are ready to start practicing.

Nurses are your primary assistants. They can filter many calls, give shots, assist in examinations, and do the administrative side of clinical work. Of course, having a nurse present while you do some examinations is essential. Many nurses want to work part time and are often willing to work for less pay because they prefer the office working environment to the hospital or private duty.

Part of running your small business is managing your personnel. Develop a set of protocols and expectations for the staff. Let them know exactly how you expect them to interact with patients and with each other. A tension-filled office is bad for everybody, and especially bad for business. Define their jobs—drawing up a job description is often a good idea—so they have no questions of what is expected of them. And stay on top of what they are doing. Have periodic reviews and staff meetings.

MARKETING YOUR PRACTICE

In addition to joining the county and state medical societies and beginning to network with physicians at the hospital, you should consider signing up with a prepaid plan. In both IPAs and PPOs, you immediately become part of a referral network.

About two months before you are ready to open your practice, place an announcement in the local papers. Let it run for about two weeks, then stop it for two weeks, and run it again for two weeks. See if you can get the hospital to help you get a picture and an article about you in the local papers. And, finally, just as you are ready to start up, hold an open house in your office for *all* the people who have helped you—from the plumber to the hospital CEO. And invite their spouses. Even the AMA now sanctions this sort of marketing.

Try other ways to market your practice. Offer to speak to local groups about your specialty. For example, if you are a cardiologist, you could speak about health and fitness to senior citizens' groups, to the local chapter of the American Heart Association, and to business groups. You can sign up with the hospital speakers' bureau. Also, consider preparing a patient information booklet covering such items as fees, appointments, and emergencies. As your patients' friends see the booklet, it becomes an advertising tool for your practice.

If you have planned carefully and allowed yourself enough time, your new practice should start up smoothly. To keep it running smoothly, you should continue to rely on the same people on whom you relied in setting it up: your attorney, your accountant, your management consultant, your banker, and your insurance representative. As your practice grows, you may consider adding a business manager and a financial adviser to the list. But through it all, remember that you are in charge, that you have chosen to be an entrepreneur as well as a physician. You cannot leave your business completely to other people. You must be actively involved in the growth and development of your practice.

Chapter XI

Moving from an Established Practice

Physicians decide to move from established practices for a variety of reasons. Often, the reasons are personal—lifestyle needs, personality conflicts on the job, job change by spouse or significant other, marriage, divorce. Just as often, the reasons are professional—career or income enhancement, more satisfactory practice style.

Some physicians decide to move because they find that lifestyle considerations they did not think were important when they took the job have overshadowed everything else. As one emergency medicine physician said, "Good, well run emergency rooms are pretty much the same everywhere in the U.S. This one is too far from our families and too far from good snow skiing. I want to go back to New England." Some move because of problems in a group or partnership. An internist is leaving her group because of the constant fights and arguments between the other two members: "They actually seem to enjoy the chaos, but I can't stand it. The office staff is tense and nervous and even takes sides. Everything is in disarray, and it's often difficult to get anything done. I want out of here." Still others leave for more intensely personal reasons. After a lengthy and nasty custody battle, which he lost, a physician called a search consultant and said, "Get me as far away from this place as I can be and still be in the United States. Everywhere I go, I'm reminded of the girls and of the fact that I'll be able to see them about twice a year."

Like their counterparts in academia and in business, people in academic and corporate medicine often find that they must move to advance professionally and financially, to "leverage" their careers. If, for example, you are an assistant professor in a program where the chairperson and tenured professors are relatively young and seem likely to stay in their positions, you will have to move if you want to be promoted or to develop a program of your own. Or if you have taken a job in the teaching program where you trained, you may have to move because your colleagues can never quite see you as a peer. An assistant professor who is widely published and respected told a search consultant, "I'm tired of being an Indian; I'm ready to be a chief. Around here, I'm still a resident—just one that's been around longer.

Often, moves involve going from a salaried position, particularly in a staff-model HMO, to private practice of some sort. After two years of experience working in an HMO, a young physician decided to move into a group practice because "the work was stifling in lots of ways. I never really developed any patient relationships, and I felt hemmed in by all the rules and regulations. Also, when I left training, I wasn't ready for the challenges of private practice. My work here was a kind of bridge between training and the real world. Now, I look forward to the challenges."

Some physicians move in the opposite direction. Tired of coping with ever-increasing paperwork and malpractice insurance and with the constant threat of HMOs eroding their practices, they move to salaried positions which relieve them of many of the problems of private practice. An internist who twice saw his practice almost cut in half by the arrival of large HMOs, took a job in institutional medicine. "I'm making just as much as I was before, and now I have pretty regular hours, set vacations, great benefits. I even get to see my kids these days, and when I tell my wife what time I'll be home for dinner, she believes me. You lose some prestige with your colleagues and credibility as a good doc, but the benefits definitely outweigh those drawbacks."

Whatever your reasons, if you do decide to move, you have to consider many of the same things you did when you were looking for your first job. Although by now you probably have a clearer picture of what you want in a job than you did when you started, you still need to look at your priorities in terms of lifestyle, professional, and financial needs, particularly your financial needs. Unless you have a salaried position in academic or corporate medicine or with an HMO, you might have to take an initial cut in income. You also need to reassess your value in the marketplace in the light of your experience.

In getting your first job, you may not have had to market yourself or to interview extensively or to negotiate a contract. Now, you may need to know how to do all these things. In discussing a candidate for a chair at a well known teaching hospital, a search consultant said,

"He wants to move, but he's a babe in the woods. He didn't have an updated CV and needed help developing one that reflected his qualifications. He showed up for his interview wearing a worn polyester suit that goes back at least 10 years. A member of the search committee described him as looking 'like someone who just fell off the turnip truck.' When I suggested as tactfully as I could that he consider a new suit, he told me he's a doctor, not a 'male model.' He's a great person and has excellent credentials, but convincing my client to hire him is going to be difficult."

Unless you have had a great deal of experience in negotiating contracts, you definitely should have an attorney help you if you are leaving an established position or practice. You need the attorney to help you determine the restrictions of your current contract that apply if you break it—such things as non-compete clauses, payment of accounts receivable, buy-out arrangements. You should have the attorney look over your new contract, or, if negotiations will be complicated, you may want the attorney to assist you in drawing up your new contract.

If you are setting up your own practice for the first time, Chapter X offers suggestions about how to get started. You should work closely with an attorney, an accountant, and a practice management consultant. When you move to another area, you should also go to a relocation specialist who understands the needs of professional people. A good relocation specialist can ease your transition by helping you see how and where your particular needs fit into the community.

If you want to move to another state, find out the licensing requirements in that state before you even interview for the job. Some states' licensing requirements are very restrictive. Some have limited reciprocity with other states and Canada. And some require that you pass their own written and oral examinations, which may be given only once or twice a year.

If you decide to set up a solo practice and are not being brought in by a hospital, make sure that you will be able to get hospital admitting privileges. Getting admitting privileges in a highly competitive area can be difficult. To discourage even more competition, some hospitals in those areas may have closed their staffs.

When they decide to move, experienced physicians must consider some things that do not usually apply to people going into their first jobs. Unless you have occurrence insurance, which you probably do not since it is so expensive that it is virtually being phased out as a form of professional liability insurance, you need to make sure you have tail insurance. If you have claims-made malpractice insurance, you are covered only while you are in your present position. Your malpractice insurance in your new position will not cover any suits that come out of your former practice and are brought against you after you leave. If you do not have tail insurance, talk to your insurance representative and your attorney to see what you can do to get it.

Another special consideration is the possibility of a sign-on bonus. If you are being recruited for a job and your potential employers or partners are eager to have you join them, you can sometimes negotiate a sign-on bonus. One young chairperson received a $15,000 bonus when she agreed to head a department at a large hospital.

Because of your professional experience, you can be much more demanding than a new physician in negotiating terms for entering a group or partnership. The terms will vary according to your special needs and priorities, but you will probably want to consider such things as buy-in, accounts receivable, authority in decision making, and administrative responsibilities.

Also, especially if you are in one of the medical or surgical subspecialties, you need to determine exactly how you will fit into the organization. Will you have your own department? Or will you be under another department? If, for example, you are an orthopedist, you will have much more autonomy and flexibility if you are in your own department than you will if you are just a member of the surgery department. You will also have more clout at budget time.

If you are moving from a private practice, you must notify your patients in writing. And you must arrange for the proper transfer of records of patients who decide to go to a new physician rather than to stay in the practice. The original records belong to you, but you must transfer at least copies of the patients' files. You can usually charge the patients for copying and mailing expenses. Failure to notify your patients and to transfer their records can be seen as abandonment—with all its legal ramifications. Again, you probably should have an attorney advise you.

Buying or selling a practice is so complicated that you should not attempt either without the professional assistance of an attorney, an accountant, and preferably a practice broker. In either case, you have to analyze the practice to determine its value in the market. To do so, look at such things as good will, accounts receivable, hard assets, and average cash flow.

If you are the seller, have a professional appraisal done. Decide if you will remain with the practice for a time, and if so, how long and how you will be compensated for your time. Also, look at what specific things you are willing to do to effect a smooth transition. If you own the building, decide if you will sell it or if you will just sell the practice and lease the space to the new physician. Decide how you will handle accounts receivable and what kind of non-compete clause you can agree to. Finally, determine not only the asking price and terms of sale but also your lowest acceptable price and acceptable alternative terms.

If you are the buyer, you job is more complicated. You need to evaluate and analyze every aspect of the practice from the staff to the demographics of the service area, from the outstanding debts and expenses to the gross and net income. You should arrange for your own inventory and appraisal of hard assets. Decide how you are willing to handle accounts receivable. Look at how the income is generated—is it fee-for-service, capitated, or mixed? If it is mixed, what are the percentages? Also, evaluate such things as the referral base, staff privileges, and goodwill. Finally, determine exactly what price and terms you can agree to.

Moving from an established practice or position is a complicated procedure. Because each move becomes more complicated and often more unsettling than the last, make sure you think through every aspect of the move when you decide to make it. Some people become so irritated in their current positions that they will agree to almost anything to get out of them. Do not. Your current irritations might fade into nothing in the face of the new irritations you could be setting yourself up for. Remember not to try to make the move on your own. Get professional advice to help you avoid problems. Then you will not have to get it to help you solve them. You know what you think of people who try to self-medicate and then come to you when they have complicated what could have been a fairly straightforward treatment.

BIBLIOGRAPHICAL ESSAY

Much of the information in this book, particularly in chapters three, four, six, seven, and eight, comes from Patricia Hoffmeir's many years of experience as a health-care and physician search consultant. Other information comes from the experiences of physicians and health-care executives. We spent the last two years interviewing hundreds of people involved in providing health-care in the United States. Because all but a few were adamant about remaining anonymous, we agreed that we would not identify any of them. We decided that their frank, and sometimes not popular, opinions were more valuable than whitewashed versions of what they were seeing and experiencing every day in medicine.

Chapter I is a survey, or summary, of what people are saying about the future of medicine. It is not intended to be definitive. As those of you in medicine know, it is possible to formulate conflicting predictions about medicine's future—depending on how you read the statistics, or on whose statistics you use. Also, medicine is changing so rapidly that some of this information may be outdated by the time the book is published. Most of the information in the chapter can be found in recent articles in newspapers such as the *Wall Street Journal* and the *New York Times,* health-care journals such as *JAMA* and *Medical Economics,* and magazines such as *Newsweek* and *U.S. News & World Report.*

For example, a discussion of the problems of practicing medicine today appeared in two different articles in the April 10, 1987, edition of the *Wall Street Journal:* "Hassles and Red Tape Destroy Joy of Job for Many Physicians" and "Dissaffection of Doctors is Discouraging Medical Students and Potential Ones." The same type of article appeared in the December 12, 1986, edition of the *New York Times:* "More Docs Look to Posts with Salaries, Report Says." On

May 8, 1987, *Modern Healthcare* contained "Physicians Leave Practice for Hospital Jobs."

More specifically, information in this chapter came from the following sources:

Flint, Austin, M.D., LL.D. *Medicine of the Future: An Address Prepared for the Annual Meeting of the British Medical Association in 1886.* D. Appleton and Company, New York, 1886. (published posthumously)

The prediction about HMO chains taking over appears in, among other places, "A New Rx for Health." *Philadelphia Inquirer.* December 15, 1985. Goldsmith's quotes are from his article about the future of medicine in *JAMA*'s January 26, 1987, issue and from his book, *Can Hospitals Survive?* Dow Jones-Irwin, Homewood, Illinois, 1981.

Articles about the disappearance of solo private practice appear in a variety of places—among them, David Nash's "Is Private Practice On Its Way Out?" *Focus.* April 15, 1987. Another typical article about the difficulties of practicing medicine in the future is "Report Predicts Hard Times Ahead" in the May 5, 1987, issue of *Hospitals.*

One article about the need for cooperation between hospitals and physicians, "Physicians say quality of care at hospitals depends on the quality of doctors—survey," appears in the May 22, 1987, issue of *Modern Healthcare.*

Christine Cassell is quoted in "Doctors Are Studying Ethics." *New York Times.* January 18, 1987.

Much of the background information for this chapter came from Paul Starr's *The Social Transformation of American Medicine.* Basic Books, Inc., Publishers, New York, 1982. It is an excellent, readable study of how American medicine has changed.

One of the places in which the figures about the growth of HMOs appear in "HMO chains grow faster than independent plans." *Hospitals.* April 5, 1986. The results of the Johnson & Higgins survey were reported in the *AHA News.* February 2, 1987. In the same issue was "Credentialling Program Planned for PPAs." The results of the Arthur Anderson survey were reported in the "a.m. Bulletin" on February 3, 1987, at the American Hospital Association's annual meeting.

A typical article about the growth of PPOs is "PPO Growth Spreads," in *Ambulatory Care,* March 1987.

Many of the figures about the supply of physicians comes from the Graduate Medical Education National Advisory Committee (GEMNAC) Summary Final Report and its 1982 update by the Department of Health and Human Services. Figures of this sort and figures about typical salaries and debts appear in a variety of places— *Wall Street Journal, New York Times, JAMA, Medical Economics, Hospitals,* United States Government statistics, to mention just a few.

Much of the information about the rehumanization of medicine comes from talks with people in medicine. And some of it comes from articles such as "The Revolution in Medicine" in the January 26, 1987, issue of *Newsweek.* That article and the one in the same issue of *U.S. News & World Report* are both interesting summaries of what has been happening to medicine in the United States in the last few years.

The merger of the city hospitals is discussed in "City Hospitals Merge to Survive" in the October 7, 1986, issue of the *Bethlehem Globe Times.* Goldsmith discusses the Rochester experiment in his January *JAMA* article.

Sturm is quoted in "Doctors Drum Up Business Success," in the September 29, 1986, issue of *Insight.* Wenneker is quoted in "Rx for Medics: More Young Doctors Shun Private Practice, Work as Employees" in the January 13, 1986, issue of the *Wall Street Journal.*

Chicago's Partnerships in Health was reported in "Eight Not-for-profits Contract to Help Care for Chicago's Poor" in the February 2, 1987, issue of the *AHA News.*

Rising medical costs were discussed in "Medical Care Costs Rose 7.7% in '86" in the February 9, 1987, issue of the *New York Times.*

Information in Chapter II comes primarily from interviews with people in medical education, from medical students and residents, and from the AMA statistics published each year in *JAMA* on numbers and types of residents. In addition, we incorporated suggestions from Anita Taylor's *How To Choose a Medical Specialty.* W. B. Saunders Company, Philadelphia, 1986.

In Chapter III, the results of the survey about how people expect doctors to look were reported in the January 2, 1987, issue of *JAMA.*

For some of the information in Chapter V, we relied on the following sources:

Gerson, J. R., and Kenneth Friendenreich. "Alternative Health Care Delivery: More Than Alphabet Soup." *Piedmont Airlines,* April 1987.

Gordon, Don. "HMOs: The Wave of the Future?" *Options,* January 1987.

McCormick, John, et al. *The Management of Medical Practice.* Cambridge, Ballinger Publishing Company, Massachusetts, 1978.

Nash, David B. Personal Interview. May 1987.

Nash, David B., editor. *Future Practice Alternatives in Medicine.* Igaku-Shoin, New York, 1987.

Tibbitts, Samuel, and Allen Manzano. *PPOs: An Executive's Guide.* Pluribus Press, Inc., Chicago, 1984.

In Chapter VI, the information about the monetary value of fellowship training was taken from George Longshore's "Choosing a Career Path: Part 1—How Much Am I Worth?" *Hospital Physician,* August 1984.

Much of the information in Chapter IX comes from interviews with attorneys, physicians, and health-care executives. And the following books provided background information on accounts receivable and guarantees:

Lewitt, Suzanne. *Physician Recruitment: Strategies That Work.* Aspen Systems Corporation, Rockville, Maryland, 1982.

McCormick, John, et al. *The Management of Medical Practice.* Cambridge, Ballinger Publishing Company, Massachusetts, 1978.

For both Chapters X and XI, we relied on information from people with many years of experience in practice management—primarily Thomas Battles and Sandra Grossman, both of Garofolo, Curtiss & Company. We also interviewed many practicing physicians and incorporated some of the advice in Yvonne Mart Fox's "How To Analyze A Practice For Sale" in the May 1987 issue of *Resident and Staff Physician.*

INDEX

Taylor, Anita, 25, 29, 35
Tibbitts, Samuel, 80

Urgent care centers (UCCs), 6, 83

Verbal commitment, 153

Women in medicine, 12, 28, 61, 100, 134
World Directory of Medical Schools, 26

Zimney, George, 28